The
Farmhouse
Diet

The Farmhouse Diet

A commonsense, no-nonsense approach to
eating healthy and healthy living. Eat the way
our grandparents and great-grandparents ate.
Sometimes the old ways are the best ways.

Warning: This is *not* a diet book . . . it's a lifestyle book.

Wm. Jay Suggs, MD

ISBN Paperback: 978-1-7378701-0-4
ISBN eBook: 978-1-7378701-1-1

Cover & Interior Design: Creative Publishing Book Design
Cover Art: Bogdan Maksimovic

To the love of my life, my wife, Elena, whose behind-the-scenes support allows me to engage in projects such as writing *The Farmhouse Diet*. To my three beautiful daughters, who exemplify womanhood. And to all the thousands of patients who have been my greatest teachers and have thus inspired me to write this book.

Contents

Preface ix

CHAPTER 1 — FOOD: Farm to Fork to Fat 1

CHAPTER 2 — Diet Science 101 19

CHAPTER 3 — Diets (Don't) Work 37

CHAPTER 4 — Your New Diet, Your New Lifestyle 49

CHAPTER 5 — Walk, Run, Race! 69

CHAPTER 6 — A Trip to the Market 77

CHAPTER 7 — Cook. Serve. Eat. Repeat. 87

CHAPTER 8 — When Food Goes Wrong 95

CHAPTER 9 — Teen Weight Loss 99

CHAPTER 10 — Nutrition for Life 103

Epilogue 115

APPENDIX 1 — Weight-Loss Surgery and
Nonsurgical Weight-Loss Devices 117

APPENDIX 2 — The Seven Habits of Highly Effective Dieting 133

APPENDIX 3 — Strategies for Dieting Success 135

Endnotes 137

About the Author 139

Acknowledgments 141

Preface

*W*arning: *This is* not *a diet book! But it is a lifestyle book.*

Most diet and nutrition books are rather thick, have hundreds of references and dozens of recipes, and dive into details that most dieters avoid reading. *The Farmhouse Diet* is only about thirty thousand words long because I wanted to produce a useful work that could easily be read in one sitting, slipped into a jacket pocket, and readily understood by a wide audience.

This book is not a scientific treatise, nor a diatribe, nor a cookbook. It is a book that you can immediately put to work for you. I hope that you enjoy reading—nay, studying—it as much as I enjoyed writing it. I hope that you savor its advice as much as I enjoy talking about nutrition and a healthy lifestyle. And I hope that if *The Farmhouse Diet* proves useful to you, and especially if it transforms your lifestyle, you will pass it on.

CHAPTER 1

FOOD: Farm to Fork to Fat

Let food be thy medicine and medicine be thy food.
—Hippocrates

Why the Farmhouse Diet?

Obesity, irritable bowel syndrome, chronic headaches, and fibro-myalgia barely existed three generations ago. So what has changed? How did our grandparents and great-grandparents eat and live? If you are fortunate enough, like me, to still have living grandparents and to have known great-grandparents (and even great-great-grandparents), you may have some insight into this question.

Have you ever looked at your teeth in the mirror? We are built with canines for tearing meat, incisors for chomping vegetables, and molars for grinding grain. We're designed to be omnivores. We're not intended to eat just meat, or just vegetables, or avoid grains, as some diets recommend. Our own mouths are telling us what we are supposed to eat. And our tummies are telling us not to eat the processed foods, simple carbs, and sugars that are a mainstay of the postmodern American diet, or *diaita* (δίαιτὰ) *Americana*, as I call it.

1

Historically, hunter-gatherers like Native Americans ate meat, fish, nuts, fruits, and vegetables. Some groups later cultivated grains such as corn and wheat. They grew potatoes and other hardy crops. Breads, ancient grains, olive oil, and dairy products were staples of the ancient Middle East. Mummified Neanderthals have been exhumed with berries, meat, and grains found in their stomachs. Archaeological evidence, as well as ancient writings such as the Bible, give us insight into how our ancestors ate. Were antediluvian early humans vegetarians, or did they also eat fish? Human societies have probably never been strictly vegetarian or vegan, but they certainly never ate as much meat as Americans do today. The Bible states that Daniel, Shadrach, Meshach, and Abednego had very healthy complexions after eating a diet of vegetables (which vegetables, grains, and starches are unknown) and avoiding the rich Babylonian diet of the royals. And it did not include potato chips and fast food. Bread, meat, and dairy have always been part of almost every culture in the world throughout history. Until recent decades, completely isolated tribes in South America and tribal people in Africa existed. They ate diets high in fruit and fiber, with little meat and, most importantly, no processed foods. These tribes also had no obesity, no colon cancer, no heart disease, and no diabetes. These societies are most comparable to ancient cultures.

The Problem of Obesity

Many of my great-grandparents were American farmers: Gillilands, Robinsons, Sidenstrickers, Carmichaels, and Pullens. There was not a hint of obesity in any of them. My great-great-grandmother, Big Mama, weighed only ninety-eight pounds and lived to be ninety-eight years old! Around the turn of the century and before the war, my grandparents worked hard and enjoyed the fruits of their labor.

They ate well. Their diets included meat, vegetables, bread, dairy, corn, beans, and grains. What they did not have were all the drive-throughs, prepackaged processed foods, and refined sugar that we consume today.

My grandparents came of age during the Great Depression. Food was often hard to come by. At that time, they did not have much meat. But they did eat a lot of beans, cabbage, corn, and grains. They had no processed food and very few commercially canned foods (although my grandmothers often did the canning themselves). Fruits were a special treat, the way desserts are for us now. They did not eat out, did not eat fast food, and did not snack. They walked almost everywhere. Riding in a car was a luxury. The kids worked in the fields while on summer break from school. There was no TV, no internet, and no video games to turn them into couch potatoes.

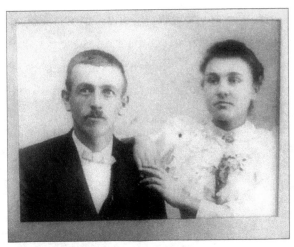

*Figure 1-1. Great-great-grandparents
in the late nineteenth century*

Old photographs tell the story of the fitness of my grandparents and great-grandparents. In their youth, they had slim waistlines.

3

However, I remember them not as trim and lithe but as pleasantly plump.

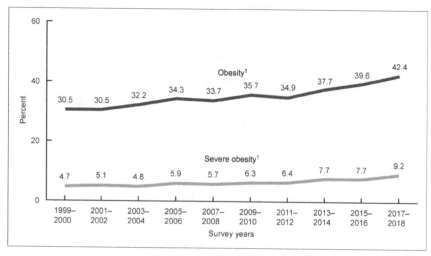

Figure 1-2. The increase in obesity through the years

After World War II, processed foods, modern cuisine, and the automobile began to have their impact on these generations, as well as on their children. Obesity began to run rampant. The jogging craze of my youth somehow missed my parents, grandparents, aunts, and uncles.

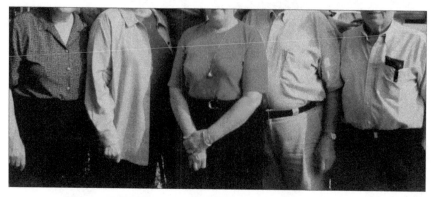

Figure 1-3. American family in the twenty-first century

Immigrants to the United States, particularly those from Asia, gain weight as they adapt to the American lifestyle and diet. This occurs even when they retain many of their traditional foods and cooking techniques. The children of immigrants from south of the border rapidly adopt the *diaita Americana* and are often overweight, if not obese. Within two generations, descendants of immigrants are plagued with obesity and weight-related diseases as much as any other American.

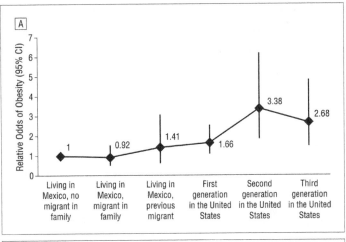

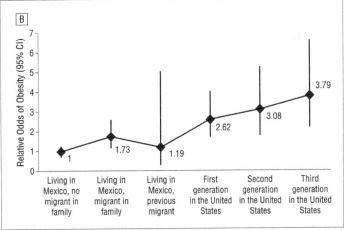

Figure 1-4. *Odds of Mexican immigrants to the United States developing obesity (top graph, men; bottom graph, women).*

To put it bluntly and unasham-
edly: How did we get so fat? Not
to be pejorative about the leading
health crisis in the United States
in the twenty-first century, but
this is a really big problem (no pun
intended). It has to be dealt with
head-on. In fact, obesity is now a
global health crisis. Who would have
thought that third-world nations,

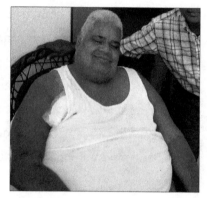

Figure 1-5. *Patient in the Dominican Republic*

even ones with 99 percent of the population living in poverty, would
now have obesity and its consequences as leading health issues? It's not
uncommon to have undernutrition, malnutrition, and overnutrition
as concurrent health crises, all within the same country.

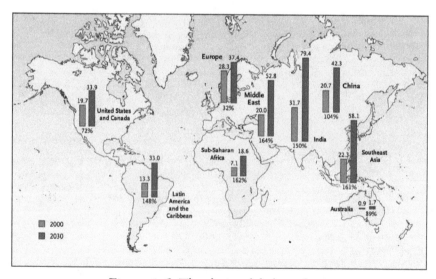

Figure 1-6. *The obesity global pandemic*

But why is being overweight or obese even a problem? Do you
believe that a balanced diet equals 50 percent healthy food and 50

percent junk food? We all know "healthy fat people." The sad truth is that over 80 percent of obese people have health problems caused by obesity. Health problems associated with obesity include the following:

Diabetes

High blood pressure

High cholesterol

Heart disease

Arthritis, including hip and knee destruction requiring joint replacement

Gout

Sleep apnea

Chronic abdominal pain

Fibromyalgia

Depression

Acid reflux

Gallstones

Higher risk of stroke

Higher risk of breast, pancreatic, uterine, and other cancers

Another interesting medical phenomenon is the risk of a disease known as biliary dyskinesia. This occurs when a patient has the symptoms of a gallbladder attack but no gallstones. The disease was nonexistent fifty years ago. Its incidence is on the rise, which almost certainly is linked to the change in American eating habits.

Teenagers needing gallbladder surgery. Clothing size 6 now being the new size 2. Seats in new stadiums now being made three inches wider than in older stadiums. Supersize fast food. Children developing diseases that you would expect in adults. Skyrocketing Social Security disability rates related to obesity.

Shocking, isn't it? Good health is linked to diet and nutrition, as well as activity. How one feels is linked to diet, nutrition, and activity. In other words, a good diet, proper nutrition, and activity are the keys to feeling good and being healthy.

Animated movie fans or folks with young children may be familiar with the movie *WALL-E*. Part of the premise of the movie is that the people who have left Earth and live on a giant space cruise ship no longer need to work or be active. They simply live for their own entertainment and unlimited consumption. All the occupants of the ship are severely obese and scoot around on little hovering lounge chairs. The most eye-opening part of the movie is when a wall displaying portraits of captains of the ship through the generations shows a progression from normal body habitus to morbid obesity. Are we destined to become like these space travelers?

Even though this book is in part about combatting the global obesity crisis, let's not confuse "being fat" with the nutrient "fat." Fat is a part of a healthy diet and should not be shunned like it has been in recent decades. We will discuss its role in a healthy, balanced diet in chapter 2.

So, to answer the question, why the Farmhouse Diet? Because, sadly, as you know, diets fail, diets are hard, and diets don't fit into our busy lives. But this is not a diet book. It's a lifestyle book. If you're ready to dramatically change your life without radically altering your life, if you're ready to change your lifestyle to a healthy lifestyle for good, if you're sick and tired of being sick and tired, then join me and millions of others in becoming healthier through better diet and nutrition.

In many ways, *The Farmhouse Diet* is a throwback to times past. Unlike other diet books, the premise of this one is that we must carefully examine history rather than relying only on the latest scientific "facts" to achieve weight loss. I always approach the newest publications on diet and weight loss with skepticism. Today's "fact" is tomorrow's laughable fallacy. This diet is not the latest fad. In fact, it's anti-fad.

When I think of healthy eating and a healthy, active lifestyle, I think of the farm. Specifically, the farmhouse where food is cooked and eaten. But the Farmhouse Diet also includes new, more health-conscious aspects. Modern society has evolved, for good or bad, in ways that our grandparents and great-grandparents could never have imagined. The way we live in the twenty-first century has to be taken into account to successfully craft a diet that becomes a lifestyle. The modern lenses of nutrition and metabolism have been used to take a new look at old ways and thus create the diet and lifestyle approaches of the Farmhouse Diet. Hopefully, you will gain a fresh perspective on healthy habits of Americans from three to four generations ago and incorporate them into your own lifestyle.

The Farmhouse Diet is not anti-fat, anti-gluten, anti-carb, anti-wheat, or anti-grain. It is a varied diet with all foods included—but in moderation. It's not judgmental about how one became overweight or obese. It focuses on healthy lifestyle choices, healthy eating, and improving one's health rather than obsessing about a weight-loss number per se. It understands that eating healthy in modern America is hard and that there are many saboteurs surrounding those who attempt to do so. The Farmhouse Diet emphasizes eating a variety of fresh fruits and vegetables, whole grains, beans, and lean meats. It de-emphasizes processed foods, prepackaged foods, and fast foods. Eating home-cooked meals with the whole family is a core value of this diet, just like it is on the farm.

It's also important not to confuse environmental causes or political causes with diet and good health. The Farmhouse Diet is primarily about achieving a healthy weight and lifestyle changes. It's not about sustainable farming, poisoning the land with pesticides, communal farming, the ozone layer, the contribution of farming to global warming, fair-trade coffee production, the national debt, income inequality, or saving Social Security. Although these may be worthy social and environmental problems to tackle, this book remains neutral on these subjects. My sole interest in writing this book is to help the reader lose weight and achieve good health. So let's get started by introducing what will be covered:

Why we're fat

Why diets don't work

Why lifestyle changes are the only way to improve weight and health

Specifics of the Farmhouse Diet

What to eat and what not to eat

Strategies for successfully maintaining your diet and lifestyle changes

Tips for cooking and exercise

What to do when you fail (and you will fail, but you can pick yourself up and press on)

The role of weight-loss surgery, weight-loss drugs, and devices to aid your weight loss

The American History of Food

Do you pick your vegetables out of the garden every day, slaughter your own pigs, wring the necks of chickens, rise early to milk the cow, or harvest your own wheat? Perhaps you go to the outdoor market every day to find fresh foods to prepare for your family in your outdoor kitchen. Or maybe you and your family set out on a daily hunt for small game, mushrooms, and wild root vegetables in the forest. Highly unlikely.

The typical American family, in contrast, will likely be found foraging in the frozen-food aisle of the grocery store, harvesting leftovers from the back of the fridge, pulling their wagon up to a drive-through, and tracking pizza preparation on an app. Hunting and gathering, farming, and outdoor markets have been replaced by the convenient grocery store, mega-mart buy-in-bulk warehouses, and assembly-line fast-food chains. Clearly, the way we produce, distribute, prepare, and even eat food has changed since the founding of America. The most dramatic changes have occurred since World War II. There are only a handful of older Americans left from the generation before the modern era of food production and consumption to tell us about the good old days.

The history of food production and consumption in the United States, especially in the eighteenth and nineteenth centuries, is fascinating. No, really. Thomas Jefferson had a vision of an America dotted with small family farms. Each family would produce its own food, with extra to sell to other people, who would engage in other pursuits, such as artisan crafting, cottage industry manufacturing, and statesmanship. Paradoxically, he and many of the founding fathers owned large plantations utilizing a slave-labor chain that produced massive quantities of basic staples such as cotton, rice, and sugar. Better planting techniques, including crop rotation and the use of natural fertilizers, were introduced. Weather almanacs, which reliably predicted the seasons' weather, improved productivity. The cotton gin, improved plows, and then tractors were among the biggest advances in the new American century. Improved methods to get products to market, such as shipping along canals, steamboats, and rail transportation, brought more food and more variety to more people. Refrigeration, canning in factories, and food preservatives were revolutionary. Before long, it was "a chicken in every pot" for Sunday dinner and a "car in every garage" to make a supermarket run. The progress since World War II has been even more impressive.

An appreciation of the changes in the process of moving food from the farm to the grocery store is not necessary to understand the evolution of food preparation, however. Our ancestors cooked on open flames or on a large fireplace hearth. Benjamin Franklin then introduced us to the use of the potbellied stove to not only heat our homes but also cook our food. Water for cooking flowed into the home rather than being carried from the well, the pump, or the creek. Rather than producing one's own staples, such as sorghum and flour, these could be purchased in a market. Over time, kitchens moved from a small building outside to the main house. In the twentieth century, as visually demonstrated in Disney World's Carousel of Progress, kitchens now had iceboxes to keep food fresh, sinks with running water, and gas or electric stoves. After World War II, a variety of food and the devices to prepare food, which were formerly available only to the rich, were now in the homes of the masses. And the growing middle class demanded yet more. In the last few decades, would any modern kitchen be considered complete without a microwave, dishwasher, and garbage disposal? In our twenty-first-century home, my wife and I now have a convection steam oven that makes the most incredibly tasty food in short periods of time.

There are many positive things to say about the modern era of food production. It has eliminated hunger and malnutrition in much of the world. Nutrition has played a vital role in decreasing infant mortality rates. Because good nutrition is the cornerstone of good health, people are living longer, healthier lives than they did two or more generations ago. Cooking and eating are now fun, not laborious or simply a means of survival. People are able to spend significantly more of their day pursuing interests not directly related to surviving to the next day. Artistic pursuits, enriching the lives of other people, and even entertainment are now not just possible but ubiquitous. Across the entire globe, twenty-first-century humans live in the wealthiest, safest period in all of human history. My great-grandparents would have thought some aspects of our modern lives ludicrous, such as the idea of owning a vacation home, racing your own race car on the weekends, or spending 76 percent of your time *not* working. Living into one's nineties and beyond seemed a remote possibility.

The same technology and practices that have made such a positive impact on our global citizenry have also fueled the obesity epidemic and its concomitant medical and social ills, such as diabetes and reduced personal productivity. The bloated, prepackaged, fast-food American lifestyle has been exported to the rest of the world. There are also growing concerns that the very food that has done so much good ultimately will prove to be hazardous to our health. The movements to produce food without the use of genetically modified organisms (GMOs), promote organic foods, and farm

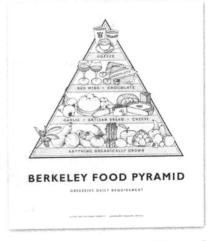

Figure 1-7. Berkeley Food Pyramid

in more environmentally friendly ways have grown exponentially. Going gluten-free, avoiding high-fructose corn syrup, and eating vegan are not only feasible endeavors but relatively easy now compared to just a decade ago.

For a vision of what healthy food production in the near future could look like, visit Epcot at Disney World in Florida. The Land Exhibit demonstrates how healthy food can be mass-produced for an increasingly more populous world using less water, less energy, and less land. Potentially, this can be done in an environmentally friendly, non-GMO, even organic fashion. But in the interest of feeding the most people the most healthy and satisfying food over the next century, we have to entertain the use of genetically modified plants and animals, nonorganic fertilizers, and people-first strategies to accomplish these goals.

The way we produce food, cook food, and eat food has changed in the last three centuries, mostly for good but also for bad. We, as a society, can continue to produce and deliver the necessary quantity of food to support a growing population and do it in such a way that we can continue to enjoy other pursuits. But we will have to start doing it in a more sustainable fashion and make food in ways that will improve health rather than worsen health. The food revolution continues.

Organic Food

Biochemically, *organic* means that the substance has carbon atoms. Really, all food is organic. Substances like rocks and plastic and even water are "inorganic." In modern times, in relationship to food, *organic* has come to mean that a food is produced without the aid of artificial fertilizers or pesticides, that animals are not given hormones or antibiotics, and that the food product is not a GMO or irradiated. The concept of non-GMO food is a bit of a fallacy, however—farmers have been genetically modifying foods through cultivation for thousands of years. Through selectively breeding animals and plants, farmers have produced higher-yield crops and herds and more nutritious foods. The first record of genetically modifying livestock comes from the book of Genesis when Jacob bred his goats to be more vigorous than his uncle Laban's, and that was almost four thousand years ago!

So, is organic food healthier? Do the lack of chemical additives and avoidance of pesticides make food better? Many people are passionate about the topic, but for weight loss and maintenance, it's not really that important. Organic food is often more expensive, and perhaps one's hard-earned dollars are better spent buying high-quality meat and fresh vegetables. Farmers markets, co-ops, specialty stores like Sprouts, and certainly your own garden can be sources of lower-cost organic foods, especially vegetables, fruits, and grains.

To assess your current diet and lifestyle choices, begin by completing the following dietary questionnaire. These questions are not designed to give you a guilt trip but to allow you to honestly assess yourself. Only with introspection and self-reflection will you be prepared to begin your weight-loss journey.

Diet and Lifestyle Questionnaire

When were you at your lowest weight and for how long?

What was your highest weight? Was it tied to an emotional event?

Have you tried a weight-loss program before? If so, how much weight did you lose?

Have you ever taken medications for weight loss? If so, which ones?

Do you have a "partner" in your weight-loss efforts?

What is your goal?

How many hours do you sleep at night?

How many minutes do you exercise or engage in physical activity each day?

What kinds of physical activity do you engage in?

What barriers are there to your engaging in physical activity?

How often do you eat out each week?

What foods do you snack on?

How many sodas or sweet beverages do you drink a day?

Do you snack after supper? Do you eat dessert?

Check all that apply:

- ❏ Eat large portions
- ❏ Eat sugary foods
- ❏ Eat fatty foods
- ❏ Use too much salt
- ❏ Eat too quickly
- ❏ Eat little to no fruit
- ❏ Skip meals
- ❏ Don't like to cook

- ❏ Skip breakfast
- ❏ Little or no exercise
- ❏ Don't drink enough water
- ❏ Eat when not hungry
- ❏ Eat fast food frequently
- ❏ Eat little to no vegetables
- ❏ Eat junk food
- ❏ Eat out a lot

CHAPTER 2

Diet Science 101

"**W**hy am I fat?" The answer is not as simple as energy in, energy out. Unfortunately, many of the diets peddled since World War II have not been based on solid science. Some have been pushed by large organizations and entities, such as the American Heart Association, the American Dietetic Association, the American Medical Association, and even the US government, despite the lack of evidence of their benefit.

Doctors and scientists, particularly in the fields of nutrition and diet, are not necessarily as smart as the public thinks. What was dogma in medicine yesterday is a dangerous fallacy today. Which raises the question: Whom should we believe?

Historical Basis of Diet Science

The link between health and diet goes back millennia. The Apostle Paul told his young protégé, Timothy, that he should drink a little wine for his stomach ailment. The use of food for ailments and the avoidance of certain foods to prevent disease were described in the Bible as well as ancient literature thousands of years ago.

In the seventeenth century, the brilliant English physician William Harvey treated one of his severely obese patients with a diet consisting almost exclusively of meat. The patient became much thinner but also suffered some unpleasant side effects—an early version of the Atkins diet, I suppose.

A few years ago, I came across an interesting book about diet used by my great-grandmother when she was a college student: *Health through Rational Diet*, written by Arnold Lorand, MD, in 1916. This book made very astute statements even before the great scientific era of molecular genetics, pharmaceutical development, and big medical research studies. Even back then, fad diets abounded. This book proposed that diet affects appearance, vigor, mind, and intelligence. It recognized the injurious effects of a "one-sided diet," such as one consisting of all rice or all meat. It stressed the importance of starch but also the importance of quality proteins, vegetables, and fruits. Dr. Lorand was almost prescient in recognizing the health benefits and utility of the soybean. Most interestingly, he warned of the unhealthiness of eating out at restaurants and was an early advocate of a form of food labeling in restaurants.

In the Victorian era and in the early decades of the twentieth century, a time when people died from eating contaminated and poorly prepared foods, the popular diet emphasized eating safe foods. Natural foods known to produce vigor, and fat, rosy cheeks were promoted. Then came the era of processed foods after World War II. Children and adults were introduced to super-sweet, premade, or easy-to-prepare junk foods. Readily available fast foods were promoted as being healthy! The average daily caloric intake of children quickly rose, and more recently, daily physical activity has declined considerably. The new phenomenon of snacking became a way of life. Children whose modern lifestyle included less healthy eating habits became the adults who continued those habits as normative.

In turn, they passed these habits on to their children, and now *they* are the unhealthy older generation.

In the past few decades, more scientific literature about diet and dieting has been published than in the previous five thousand years combined. Even more books and essays have been written about dieting. Although modern society has orders of magnitude more knowledge, there is less wisdom about what to put in our bodies. The best chance that society has in achieving good health and healthy weight is to consider the science as well as the history of diet. My hope is that this book will give you the intellectual tools to synthesize the most pertinent facts and then craft a diet and new lifestyle that work for you.

One's Proper Weight

It would be appropriate to ask why we are well in to chapter 2 before even addressing the question of what is a normal weight. That is a tricky question whose answer has changed over time. The most common and easiest method for determining one's proper weight is by calculating body mass index. Body mass index, or BMI, is calculated by dividing weight in kilograms by height in meters squared ($BMI = kg/m^2$). Unless you are brilliant at math, the easiest way to determine your BMI is to find a calculator on the internet (such as at www.cdc.gov/healthyweight/assessing/bmi/index.html) or plug your metrics into an app. Figure 2-1 demonstrates normal and overweight/obese BMIs.

For many decades, differentiating normal, underweight, overweight, and obese weights was based on the Metropolitan Life insurance tables. Where you fell in the table was also based on whether you had a small, medium, or large skeletal frame. Unfortunately,

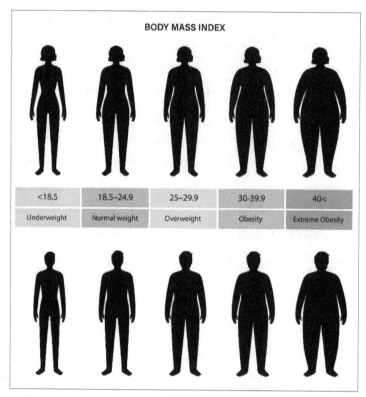

Figure 2-1. Measuring obesity in terms of body mass index

these tables are not the best method for determining normal weights. Perhaps the most accurate method for determining obesity is measuring one's body fat percentage. This can be done by weighing in water or measuring impedance with a special body composition analysis machine. The devices for making those measurements are neither readily available nor convenient. For now, the most widely accepted method used by doctors, scientists, writers, and dieters to determine obesity is to use BMI.

Another reason that the question of what is a normal weight is tricky is that the concept of "normal" versus "overweight" or "obese" differs among different races and social groups. Over time, an overall higher weight and degree of fatness has been generally accepted in society compared to generations past. Also, we must consider the distribution of body fat, that is the gynecoid (pear) versus android (apple) shapes. Twenty pounds of extra fat in the gut has more deleterious health effects than twenty pounds well distributed on the thighs and buttocks.

Ultimately, the best way to determine if you are obese is to assess the presence of disease caused or worsened by obesity; or, of limitations in mobility, exercise, or lifestyle because of excess weight. Also, a trend of increasing weight over time is a red flag. These factors are more important than a number or calculation per se.

Freshman Biochem, Sophomore Physiology

Nutrients are classified as macronutrients, which the body needs in large quantities, and micronutrients, which the body needs in small quantities. Protein, carbohydrates, and fats are macronutrients. Vitamins, minerals, and trace elements are micronutrients. All of them, even the tiny ones you might never have heard of, like manganese and molybdenum, are important for your metabolism. Protein has the lowest caloric density, and fat has the highest. Water is essential for metabolism, not just for staying hydrated. Oils are fats, dairy is fat and protein, sugar is a type of carbohydrate, and fiber is a form of complex carbohydrate. When determining parameters for weight loss and maintenance, diets focus on the macronutrients protein, fat, and carbohydrate. However, all macronutrients and micronutrients—and water—are important.

Fat storage occurs in both the liver and the subcutaneous tissue deep to the skin. Fat also surrounds the organs in the abdomen and can even build up around the heart. Sugars and carbohydrates that are not immediately used for energy are turned into fat. When carbohydrates are burned up, your metabolism turns to fat for fuel. The metabolism turns to proteins for fuel when carbs and fats are depleted. There are ways to maximize these physiologic facts to optimize weight loss.

Hormones play a major role in obesity, where fat is deposited, and success in weight loss. One key to success is to maximize these hormones' influence on your weight loss. Ghrelin, also known as the "hunger hormone," shoots up when one is dieting or in starvation mode. It is made in the stomach. Ghrelin promotes appetite and fat deposition. Leptin, which is produced in fat cells, is an important obesity regulatory hormone and is also known as the "satiety hormone." Obese individuals have too much leptin, and they can even develop a resistance to its effects. Leptin is the opposite of ghrelin. When one loses body fat, leptin levels fall. This can trigger food cravings and, therefore, increases in weight. So leptin can sabotage your diet efforts.

There are several other hormones that influence obesity and weight loss, some of which we don't fully understand. Despite all that we know about how these hormones work, especially ghrelin and leptin, medical scientists still have not discovered how to manipulate them for a truly effective weight-loss drug. However, the types of food you eat, when you eat, and avoiding hunger can suppress the hunger hormone, ghrelin, and maximize the satiety hormone, leptin.

Water

Water is often forgotten as an essential element of good nutrition. It is just as important as protein, fats, and carbohydrates. Without water, no life exists. Without safe, fresh water, human life cannot exist.

Drinking plenty of water is important for staying hydrated as well as for keeping your metabolism running. Drinking lots of water is a behavior that is associated with better weight control. You don't have to drink fancy mineral water, protein water, or vitamin water. My personal favorite is "agua fría" . . . cold, clean tap water. Keeping bottled water handy, or your own reusable water bottle, is a habit that not only keeps you hydrated but also helps curb the desire for sugary beverages and snacks. Whether drinking liquids during meals or between meals, choose water over sodas, juices, and alcohol. If you'd like some additional flavor, add a low-calorie flavoring, such as Crystal Light or a splash of lemon. Adding fresh berries and mint to your water is another way to liven it up.

Fiber

Dietary fiber is important for avoiding constipation, lowering levels of bad cholesterol, and preventing colon cancer and diverticular disease. Fiber is a low-calorie-density choice and makes one more satisfied than high-calorie-density processed foods and snack foods. Foods packing the fiber punch have nutritional value and will leave you feeling satiated much longer than foods low in fiber and poor in nutritional value. Many yummy vegetables, fruits, cereals, and grains are high in fiber as well as low in sugar and carbs. Eating more fiber is a key to weight-loss success.

Vitamin Supplements

With a varied, healthy diet such as the Farmhouse Diet, you should get all the essential macronutrients, micronutrients, and trace elements that you need. However, it's usually recommended by physicians that older adults, even those with an excellent diet, take a daily adult multivitamin. Although the jury is out on how important it is to take vitamins, go with the recommendation of your doctor.

All multivitamins should be "complete." Make sure that the vitamin contains thiamine, folate, iron, and zinc. Some vitamins, especially chewables and gummies, leave out thiamine because of its bad taste. However, thiamine is critical to vision, the ability to walk, and nervous system function. Some vitamins leave out iron. Vitamins should have all fat-soluble vitamins, including A, D, E, and K. Trace elements that look like they are straight out of the periodic table should also be listed near the bottom of the ingredients label. Women should also take extra calcium, and premenopausal women often need extra iron supplements to prevent anemia. Pregnant women should be on a prenatal vitamin.

Vitamin D, which, like calcium, is critical to good bone health, is often deficient in otherwise healthy people. Because the body can synthesize vitamin D but needs sunlight to do so, this may have something to do with Americans now spending most of their time indoors and not working outside. Vitamin B12, which is important for having energy and preventing anemia and problems with the nervous system, is a common deficiency.

Examples of complete multivitamins include One a Day, Centrum, Nature Made, Alive!, Flintstones Complete, and any bariatric multivitamin. Generic, store-brand versions of these are usually just as good but less expensive. Because vitamins are not regulated by the US Food and Drug Administration (FDA), as medications are, you may not be getting the nutrients you think you are in a particular brand of vitamin. Carefully check the bottle. You can have more confidence that the amounts of vitamins and minerals listed on the label are accurate and that the ingredients are of the highest quality if you choose a vitamin supplement that is certified by the US Pharmacopeia, or USP.

Calcium comes in the form of calcium citrate and calcium carbonate. Many experts believe that calcium citrate is superior to calcium carbonate, which is cheaper, but there is scientific evidence that the superiority of one type of calcium over the other depends on one's genetics. More important than the type of calcium is that you actually take it. Calcium citrate and calcium carbonate are absorbed differently by the gut, so pay attention to what the label says about when you should take them. Don't take them at the same time that you take the multivitamin.

Some diet plans push taking large quantities of vitamins to lose weight. Taking vitamins rather than making changes to protein, carbs, and other nutrient intake is counterproductive. Megadoses of vitamins could actually be harmful. Vitamins are important, but these diet plans focus on only one aspect of a healthy diet and lifestyle rather than addressing all necessary components.

Herbal supplements and other dietary supplements in little bottles and pillboxes marketed as weight-loss adjuncts are also not recommended. These substances are not medications and are not regulated by the FDA. Some may be harmful. Please do not take these.

VITAMINS

Physicians often recommend that middle-aged and older adults take an adult multivitamin and calcium supplement daily. Some folks need extra B12, vitamin D, and iron. For the rest of us, eating a healthy diet like the Farmhouse Diet should get us all the vitamins, minerals, and trace elements that we need. There are a variety of complete, lower-cost vitamins on the market.

So what is a complete multivitamin? It should have everything, including but not limited to thiamine (vitamin B1), biotin, B12, vitamin D, zinc, selenium, B6, vitamin A ... everything. Many chewable or gummy vitamins leave out thiamine or other essential vitamins and minerals. Check your vitamin to make sure it says "complete" or "multivitamin" and is designated for adults, not children.

Vitamin patches do not work. Physicians have seen severe vitamin deficiencies in patients using such patches. Take a good-quality oral multivitamin.

Biscuit Poisoning

Carbohydrates are turned into fat by the liver. Since the 1960s, Americans have reduced their total daily fat intake substantially but replaced it with carbs. And then some—in many cases, a few hundred calories a day more in carbs. Most of these extra carbs are in the form of processed foods and junk foods, not natural starchy foods and vegetables. *All* carbs are not bad, but the wrong kinds are. All carbs are not created equally. Simple sugars and simple carbs, such as processed wheat and potatoes, are less healthy. Complex carbohydrates, such as those found in whole grains and vegetables, are healthier.

Insulin is a driver of weight gain. Any new diabetic who just started insulin or even oral diabetes medicines will confirm that this is true. Insulin is released from the pancreas in reaction to carbohydrate intake. The insulin levels spike too quickly when one eats sugars or simple carbs. This is unhealthy. Insulin causes your metabolism to convert excess carbs to fat and also prevents your body from mobilizing this stored fat for energy. Insulin is slowly released from the pancreas when one eats complex carbs. This is healthy. Eating protein with carbs also helps smooth out the insulin release. Of note, there are some newer diabetic medications that are being used for weight loss. See the section on weight-loss medication in chapter 3.

The glycemic index is a measure of how quickly blood-sugar levels and, consequently, insulin rise in response to the ingestion of a particular type of carbohydrate. Most vegetables, meats, and complex carbs have a low glycemic index. Processed foods and those full of sugar or simple carbs, like biscuits, have a high glycemic index. In general, foods with a low glycemic index are better for you than those with a high glycemic index. However, this is a bit trickier than a simple list of low-glycemic-index foods because one also has to consider how much of that food (by weight or mass) one eats. Thus, the glycemic load has better applicability for determining what's better to eat. Watermelon has a high glycemic index but a low glycemic load and is actually very healthy. Dried apricots have a low glycemic index but actually possess quite a bit of sugar.

Gluten is not the great evil that those consumed with current health fads believe it to be. Gluten is a protein that is found in wheat, barley, oat, and rye. It causes inflammation in patients with celiac sprue. This leads to abdominal pain, diarrhea, and weight loss. Celiac sprue affects approximately one in two hundred people. It is a truly bad disease. Other folks may have some degree of gluten sensitivity. For the rest of us, gluten is not the problem as much as the other properties of the foods that contain gluten. Most processed foods, breads, and foods in boxes contain wheat gluten, but they are also full of simple carbs and sugars and have a high glycemic index. People who lose weight and feel better on a gluten-free diet do so because they are cutting out processed foods and simple carbs, not because they are cutting out gluten per se.

Wheat, the primary ingredient of breads, pastries, pasta, and even most snack foods, has been transformed over the millennia through the process of hybridization. The wheat, or *Triticum*, flour that our grandmothers and great-grandmothers used is different from what modern people use. In the late nineteenth and twentieth centuries, wheat was genetically transformed to be more easily grown and have better baking qualities. The taste of bread is different than it was hundreds of years and even decades ago. Although this transformation into modern wheat has enabled the world to be fed, it may have come at the cost of our health. The ancient einkorn and emmer wheats that our ancestors ate in prehistoric and Biblical times had greater nutritional value than the hybridized variety of wheat that we eat today.

White rice is a mainstay of the traditional Asian diet. But it was not always this way. Progress in the industrialization of foodstuffs brought a conversion from the unpolished, brown form of rice to white, or polished, rice. White rice has a much longer shelf life and is less likely to be ruined or eaten by pests than brown rice. Until recently, Chinese, Indian, Japanese, Filipino, and other Asian cultures did not have rates of overweight or obesity comparable to those in the United States. But they are catching up in the global obesity epidemic. This correlates with the increase in the consumption of less healthy white rice. In general, Asians' (especially Indians') health does not tolerate being overweight, not to mention obese. They especially do not tolerate visceral (belly) fat.

Protein

Protein is good. Protein is tasty. Protein is a low-calorie-density nutrient compared with carbohydrates and has approximately 40 percent of the calorie density of fats. Of course, it's possible to eat too much protein, but this is rarely a problem in healthy individuals. Patients with chronic renal failure are usually kept on a lower-protein diet by their nephrologists. Protein supplements can be useful for achieving initial weight loss, as in Phase 1 of the Farmhouse Diet, as well as in the maintenance of weight, such as in Phase 3 of the Farmhouse Diet. Consider a protein shake in lieu of a meal for breakfast or lunch. You can add quality protein powder to a liquid, such as water or skim milk, to make your own shake or smoothie. Or you can buy a ready-made shake or a powder requiring only water.

Protein supplements should be made of high-quality whey protein. Other forms of protein, such as those from plant sources, have less of the building blocks necessary for building muscle and maintaining good nutrition. Powders and shakes should have very little added sugar. Look for powders that say "100 percent whey" or "whey protein isolate." Unjury, Premier Protein, SlimFast, Boost, Carnation Instant Breakfast with high protein, and Muscle Milk are examples of quality commercially available protein shakes. Look for 15 to 30 g of protein per serving, less than 15 g of sugar for shakes, and less than 5 g of sugar for protein powder.

The Low-Fat Fallacy

Great harm to public health has occurred in the last fifty to sixty years with the war on fat and our love affair with sugars and simple carbs. Excess carbohydrates not immediately used for your body's fuel are converted to fat. This causes obesity, diabetes, high blood pressure, and heart disease.

Did you know that saturated fat does not cause heart disease? You heard right. New scientific evidence turns the dictum of the recent past on its head and suggests that the standard diet prior to the 1970s—rich in meat, eggs, and cheese—was healthier than the contemporary diet promulgated by "authorities." In fact, the dietary guidance issued by the American Diabetes Association, American Heart Association, and the US Department of Agriculture has probably led to more deaths from stroke, cancer, and heart disease than would have occurred if no advice were given at all.

Fat is not the enemy. Animal fat is also not the enemy. High-fructose corn syrup is the enemy. Simple sugars, processed sucrose, and high-fructose corn syrup are as addictive as drugs. Processed wheat flour is also problematic, but whole grains are not. Natural sugars, such as those found in fruits, are different. They are not unhealthy. But don't confuse fruit and fruit juice, with the latter having few redeeming qualities.

There are many dangers in having an unbalanced, high-fat, very high-protein, even ketogenic diet. These diets are impossible to maintain in the long run, with expected weight rebound when introducing carbs back into the diet. Diets that promote a state of ketosis lead to serious health risks. In medicine, we see ketosis as a dangerous thing. When patients with diabetes have ketoacidosis and ketones in the urine, it is a bad thing; they often end up in the intensive care unit or even in a coma.

Genetics and Metabolism

It's the age-old issue of genes versus lifestyle. Why do some people seem to eat everything they want, but others just look at a muffin and gain weight? The sad truth is that our genes have more to do with obesity and diet failure than any other factor. Which raises the question: Why should you continue to read this book rather than plop yourself on the couch with a bag of chips if it is true that genes are the most important determinant of obesity?

The reason is that lifestyle is also important. Twin studies often shed light on the nature-versus-nurture debate. Several studies of identical twins raised in two different households found big differences in obesity between the twins, meaning genetics isn't the only factor. Even twins who are raised together but live apart as adults can have significant differences in weight. The good news is that we are not totally slaves to our genetics. The bad news is that if you're the fat twin, then you're not the skinny twin.

Our genes predispose us to our body habitus. Our genes also predispose us to certain illnesses, such as diabetes, heart disease, and cancer. But our genes are not the sole determinant. They are just the framework. Although it is more work for some of us, we are not cursed to be obese and unhealthy because of our genes. We have to work with what we are given. This is where a healthy diet and lifestyle, as found in *The Farmhouse Diet*, become important.

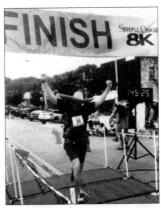

Figure 2-2. "*It's not that diabetes, heart disease, and obesity runs in your family . . . It's that no one runs in your family!*"—*Tony Robbins*

As hinted at earlier in this chapter, the location of body fat has important health implications. The two types of obesity are the android, male, type and the gynecoid, or female, type. *Android* is also synonymous with an "apple" shape and *gynecoid* with a "pear" shape. Don't let the terms fool you. Women can have an android shape, and some men can have a gynecoid shape. Because the android shape is due to greater percentages of visceral fat, or fat around and in the abdominal organs, such as the liver and omentum, it is more likely to cause metabolic syndrome. Metabolic syndrome is the deadly triad of diabetes, hypertension, and high lipids/cholesterol. Thus, a person who is forty pounds overweight with an android shape is less healthy than a person who is forty pounds overweight with a gynecoid shape. Whereas it is very important for that person with the android shape to lose weight, the gynecoid-shaped person may tolerate that extra forty pounds just fine.

There is a clear association between obesity and an increased risk of certain cancers. This includes the risk of breast, pancreatic, and uterine cancers. In fact, most cancers seem to occur more often in obese people.

Resting Your Metabolism

The proper amounts of sleep, rest, and stress reduction are important in achieving weight loss and maintenance. Less than seven hours of sleep per night or fitful sleep and high stress are associated with higher weight. Not enough sleep and rest, combined with too much stress, will make it difficult to properly lose weight. If you are the type of person who loses weight during periods of stress, when your situation improves, you may put the weight back on. Most people, however, deal with stress by eating low-quality food. This, of course, results in weight gain.

Is intermittent "resting" of your metabolism through fasting good or bad for weight loss? Most people throughout history fasted for twelve hours per night. Traditional American farmers fasted overnight, then would often eat a light predawn meal of coffee and Scottish or steel-cut oatmeal. A bigger midmorning breakfast full of protein and fat, like bacon and eggs, would follow. The concept of intermittent fasting as a diet is covered in chapter 3, and as mentioned there, it may have merit but requires more study.

Exercise, on the other hand, has a critical impact on your metabolism. It can increase your metabolism, create muscle, burn fat, and strengthen your heart. The effects of focusing your mind and relieving stress are also well known. See chapter 5 for more on exercise.

"QUESTION AUTHORITY"

This was the mantra when I was a young man in college, and it still holds true. Don't accept diet dictums that have failed you in the past. A seemingly authoritative television commercial with well-known celebrities or a flashy book cover by Dr. Know-It-All, MD, should not be taken at face value. You must investigate what works for you. The proof is in the results—in pounds lost, exercise goals met, smaller clothing sizes, and improved health. The ultimate proof is in maintaining a healthy weight and lifestyle and being able to get back on track when you slip up.

CHAPTER 3

Diets (Don't) Work

New ≠ good; old ≠ obsolete.

One diet tells us that wheat is the source of all evil, yet another tells us to eat only grains and potatoes. One authority tells us to eat only meat and fat, whereas another pushes a low-fat or vegan lifestyle. Many eschew eggs, fried food, dairy, and fruits. In other words, popular diets often give contradictory advice. What seems like the dietary answer to all our health problems becomes anathema a few years later. How can a reasonable, well-informed person possibly separate the fact from the fiction in making healthy diet and lifestyle choices?

To aid in this endeavor, in the following sections, I describe several currently popular diets, as well as their benefits and drawbacks.

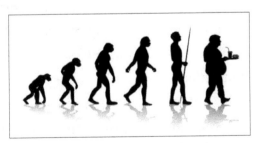

Figure 3-1. The "evolution" of modern man

Weight Watchers

This commercial diet, now known as "WW," has been around, and moderately successful, for decades. It is beneficial for many people, but some find it difficult to comply with, especially men. It utilizes a point system, in which all foods are assigned points based on calories, satiety, and other factors. No foods are off-limits per se, including sweets, carbs, and processed foods. In the past, this diet was very carb heavy and fat avoidant. All calories, no matter the source or metabolic effect, are treated equally. This severely limits the success of the Weight Watchers diet. Most patients lose only a few pounds. Long-term success is dependent on staying on Weight Watchers for a lifetime. Hope you have a lot of memory on your smartphone to keep track of decades' worth of points!

The great strength of Weight Watchers is the coaching and accountability components of this diet system. Not only does one keep careful track of food intake, but one also meets in groups and with individual coaches. In this regard, it is similar to and perhaps even more effective than undergoing behavioral counseling for weight loss.

The New Atkins Revolution

This diet has great results initially, but it is very difficult to maintain as a lifestyle. Side effects such as gastrointestinal ailments and gout are problematic. Dr. Atkins was an early pioneer in recognizing the health problems associated with the low-fat, high-carb diets being peddled by "big nutrition."

In later years, Dr. Atkins made some changes to his diet that stressed the low-carb benefits more than the high-fat and high-protein approach per se. Some of the recipes in his last edition are very tasty.

Additional changes were made in the diet protocol over the years by doctors after Dr. Atkins to include some carbs, vegetables, fiber, and more variety. With the introduction of these changes, the New Atkins Diet may be more doable. However, this diet's food options are still rather restrictive.

Paleo Diet

Paleo is good for many folks, but its philosophical underpinnings are flawed. It's based on the premise that during the Paleolithic era more than ten thousand years ago, our ancestors ate only healthy natural foods like fish, lean meat, fruits, and nuts. The way it's described, cavemen pranced around all day living a bohemian lifestyle! Clearly, the historical facts don't support this. Ancient people were ravaged by disease and did not live to be very old.

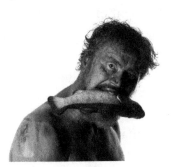

There are many benefits to the Paleo diet, like avoiding processed foods and emphasizing lean meats and vegetables. However, the Paleo diet focuses too much on meat and may be too expensive for many people. It does not allow grains or legumes. The science behind this is poor at best. Contrary to the premise of the Paleo diet, we were made to ingest grains and beans. They form a healthy part of any diet. Furthermore, as with any diet, this diet would need to be a permanent part of your lifestyle. Are you prepared to never have bread or a potato again?

South Beach Diet

The South Beach diet is a Mediterranean type of diet. It is neither high protein nor low fat, but it is mostly low carb. It was designed primarily to promote heart health more than weight loss. It avoids most animal fats, which are rich in saturated fats, and in the first phase, it avoids grains. In later phases, grains, beans, breads, and legumes are allowed. In this respect, it's very different from the Paleo, keto (discussed next), and Atkins diets. This diet relies heavily on the glycemic index to determine which foods are acceptable and which

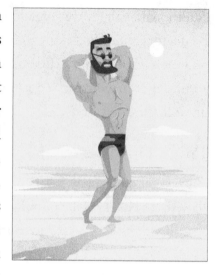

ones are not. Lean proteins, vegetables, and fiber are emphasized. Processed foods are a no-no. The South Beach diet is one of the easiest to adhere to, but the results are highly dependent on how strict the dieter is in adhering to the rules. Overall, it's a reasonable diet, but the results are highly variable.

Keto Diet

In most regards, the keto diet is like the original Atkins diet. It is a very low-carbohydrate, high-protein, and high-fat diet that sends one into a state of ketosis, in which fats and ketones, rather than carbohydrates, are burned for fuel. Fats make up 75 percent or more of the diet. Many healthy vegetables and legumes are excluded from this diet. Almost all fruits are excluded. Metabolically, ketosis can actually be dangerous. Normal, healthy folks can end up wasted, metabolically depleted, in kidney failure, and in the intensive care unit. Originally, the ketonic diet was developed as a treatment for epilepsy, and it was never intended to treat obesity. People with diabetes, kidney disease, heart disease, and other medical conditions are at even higher risk for being hospitalized while on the keto diet. Some of the diets mentioned in this chapter have been around for a long time and will continue to be popular. The keto diet, however, is a fad that is destined for the waste bin of history because it is difficult to maintain as well as for its potential for adverse health effects.

Mayo Clinic Diet

Contrary to popular belief, for most of the Mayo Clinic's storied history, there was no "Mayo Clinic diet." Recently, however, solid nutritional advice that Mayo was giving to its patients and the public has been formalized into an actual diet plan. Overall, it's easy to adhere to, but it may underemphasize protein intake and be a bit too liberal with simple carbs and sweets. This diet does not depend on counting calories or carbs or fats and instead issues general guidelines for changing your lifestyle.

Intermittent Fasting

Fasting has been a part of religious as well as health practices for thousands of years. As a weight-loss strategy, it is the latest fad to hit the market. Much of the "science" behind its theory is altering insulin metabolism. There are a variety of ways to do this, but all involve alternating fasting days with "feasting" days. Fasting days may have zero caloric intake or be equivalent to a very low-calorie diet. The dieter may skip breakfast or be limited to just one meal per day. Scientifically, this diet has not been well studied. The jury is out as to its long-term efficacy and safety, particularly in patients with diabetes and heart disease.

Vegan and Vegetarian Diets

Vegan and vegetarian diets are often very high in simple carbs and simple sugars. There are even specific diets that recommend eating lots of potatoes and rice. It is not unusual to see overweight and obese vegans in America now because they eat a lot of simple carbs and processed foods to avoid animal proteins. Vegetarian diets can be healthy if eggs and dairy are included and if vitamin and mineral supplements are taken as well. In fact, the Farmhouse Diet can be easily adapted for vegetarians. The belief that all dairy is bad for you, even if just applied to adults, is clearly wrong, both historically and based on scientific evidence (unless you have lactose intolerance or dairy allergies, of course). The risks of poor nutrition, anemia, and vitamin deficiencies are concerns with a vegan diet. Many vegans choose this diet more for philosophical or political reasons than for health reasons. I do not recommend a vegan lifestyle for those interested in weight loss and weight maintenance; it's more difficult to ensure adequate nutrition when so many foods are restricted, and a vegan diet may consist of too many carbs.

Commercial Diets with Prepackaged Foods or Shakes

Diets that offer prepacked convenience foods and shakes are very expensive, often high in carbs, and not sustainable as a lifestyle. Nutrisystem, Jenny Craig, Atkins, the South Beach Diet, SlimFast, and OPTIFAST are well-marketed examples of these types of diets. Who really thinks they can eat food that comes in little boxes in the mail or drink all their meals out of a glass for their entire lives? That's not a lifestyle. That's an aberration. The Farmhouse Diet emphasizes fresh foods and preparation of your own meals at home, as well as sustainable lifestyle choices.

FOOD FALLACIES AND FALSEHOODS

Prehistoric peoples ate lean meat and vegetables and did not eat grains.

Organic is better for weight and health than nonorganic.

Fat is bad and causes heart disease.

Eggs are bad for you.

Sugary candy is better than fatty foods.

All carbs are bad.

A calorie equals a calorie.

Simple calorie reduction equals weight loss.

All meat is bad.

All dairy is bad.

Why can't you just eat less and lose weight?

OTHER MISTAKES

Avoidance of grains and beans

Eating too much fat and too much protein

Diabetic diets, which actually make the problem worse

All-vegan diets

Ketosis

Butter/fat substitutes, such as margarine, and trans fats

So, is there any hope? Could it be that with decades of scientific research on diet and nutrition, not only are we no better off, but we are now in worse shape than ever in history? The common link between all these diets is that they often rely on radical, difficult-to-comply-with strategies that won't translate into long-term lifestyle changes. They are not natural solutions. Inadequate weight loss is one problem with conventional diets. The worse problem is that when one stops the diet, the weight comes back on—oftentimes even more weight than one lost on the diet! That's why permanent lifestyle change is critical. Now that I've trashed just about every popular diet because of poor long-term weight loss, safety issues, and compliance difficulty, what's left?

The answer lies in going back in time to investigate what kept our grandparents and great-grandparents healthy and svelte. History and current nutritional science are both equally important in this endeavor.

Weight-Loss Drugs

As you well know, dieting is hard. Most people need assistance, and that may come in the form of weight-loss drugs. Although they're not for everyone, they have their place. Contraindications due to certain medical problems or interactions with other drugs are primary considerations before starting a weight-loss drug. Patients taking benzodiazepines, psychotropic drugs, neurological drugs, chronic-pain medications, and some diabetes medicines may not be able to take weight-loss drugs.

In general, drugs can only be used temporarily, either until one's weight-loss goal has been achieved or weight loss plateaus. Some drugs can now be used for maintenance. However, there's always a price to pay when using weight-loss drugs, which may include side effects as well as serious complications. In other words, these drugs have the potential to be dangerous, addictive, and ineffective. They should only be prescribed after a thorough evaluation by a physician. This will likely include blood work, an electrocardiogram (ECG), and other testing. A consultation with a dietitian or other nutritional counselor is a must. Of course, drugs should only be used in combination with serious diet, exercise, and lifestyle changes. Without those changes, the medications are ineffective.

Weight-loss drugs can be very effective in patients who've had weight-loss surgery and subsequently regain weight. Patients who are overweight or mildly obese will have a higher success rate than those who are moderately or severely obese in terms of the percentage of extra weight that they lose.

Saxenda

Also known by its generic name, liraglutide, this is the same drug as Victoza. It is a diabetes drug that has been applied to weight loss. It works by suppressing appetite and increasing satiety, leading to decreased caloric intake. It is an injectable drug that is self-administered daily.

Qsymia

Qsymia, a combination of phentermine and topiramate, works by suppressing appetite, increasing satiety, and altering the taste of food. It is intended for patients with a body mass index (BMI) $\geq$ 30 or a BMI $\geq$ 27 with one obesity-related comorbidity. Qsymia is a capsule taken daily.

Contrave

Contrave is a combination of naltrexone and bupropion (Wellbutrin). It works not only by suppressing appetite but also by reducing cravings. The naltrexone component is used for treating opiate addiction, but in combination with bupropion, it acts as an appetite suppressant. It is for patients with a BMI ≥ 30 or a BMI ≥ 27 with one obesity-related comorbidity. This pill is taken once or twice daily.

Adipex

Also known as the generic drug phentermine, Adipex has been around for a while. It works by suppressing appetite. Formerly, it was sold as the combination drug fen-phen, which was pulled off the market in the 1990s due to the complication of heart-valve damage. The "phen" part (phentermine), however, has remained on the market. Phentermine has mild addictive potential and is not for long-term use.

Diabetes Medicines

Drugs to treat diabetes, such as metformin and Trulicity, have been utilized by some physicians in an "off-label" fashion as weight-loss drugs. However, the results in most studies are disappointing, and in general, these medications are not recommended as frontline treatments for obesity.

Realistic expectations are critical for achieving success with weight-loss drugs. A 10 percent reduction in total body weight would be a smashing success. Keeping off 5 percent of total body weight long term would be successful. Of course, this raises the question: Why even use weight-loss drugs? For many people, however, this is meaningful weight loss and just what they need to feel better and be healthier.

It can't be emphasized enough that weight-loss drugs should only be used in conjunction with other therapies. There are no magic pills. Lifestyle changes, healthy eating, and exercise are the cornerstones of weight loss. For some patients, adding an intragastric balloon or other weight-loss device, and perhaps even considering weight-loss surgery, may be their recipe for success; these options are discussed in Appendix 1.

CHAPTER 4

Your New Diet, Your New Lifestyle

What this diet is:

Lifestyle change

Common sense

Something that you can stick to

Delicious and satisfying

What this diet is not:

Faddish

Demanding that one be organic, gluten-free, grain-free, or vegan

Impossible to do long term

Expensive

Radical

Keys to diet success:

The diet must be realistic and achievable.

Lifestyle changes must be reasonable and doable.

Follow a daily eating plan.

Exercise regularly and intensely.

Improved health and fitness are more important than a number.

Maintain the weight and level of fitness that you worked so hard to achieve.

The Farmhouse Diet has three phases, which are described in detail in this chapter, designed to help you achieve your weight-loss goals and maintenance of weight. These phases, if done correctly, will set you up for long-term success.

Phase 1: Induction

This is the hardest part of the Farmhouse Diet, and it will require willpower and attention to the details of the diet. This phase is two weeks long. If it is too tough, it is OK to end the induction phase early. But if you can stick to it, it will really jump-start your weight loss. Men should expect to lose five pounds in the first week of Phase 1, and women should lose around five pounds in the first two weeks. Weight loss will slow down after that.

This is not a calorie-counting diet. It is based on carefully selecting the types of food in your diet, avoiding problematic foods, and maximizing weight loss with exercise. Accountability and getting back on track when you fail are essential elements.

In this phase, you will eliminate certain foods. It is important to eliminate all refined sugar. Pretty quickly, you will find out if you have a sugar addiction. Likewise, you may have an addiction to simple carbs, such as potato- and corn-based processed snack foods. After coming off simple carbs and sugars, your blood sugar may transiently drop. You may feel awful and experience dumping syndrome. Symptoms of dumping syndrome include nausea, sweating, shakes, weakness, and even abdominal pain. Avoid the temptation to treat your symptoms with more carbs or sugar. That will cause this vicious cycle to persist. A little caffeine may ameliorate some of those symptoms.

OPTIONAL

Another option for Phase 1 is to begin with a liquid protein diet for one to two weeks. Basically, one would substitute a protein drink for a meal. Do at least two meals a day this way, and all three meals if you have the willpower. Otherwise, one meal could be a healthy meal of solid food that still fits the Phase 1 criteria. You can make the protein shake yourself from scratch, make it from a powder, or drink a premade shake. See the section on protein in chapter 2 for a list of suggested protein supplements.

In Phase 1, you must eliminate bread, potatoes, pasta, and rice. Even whole-grain bread and pasta, as well as brown rice, are out. Carbs are OK, just not during the induction phase. Good substitutes for these food staples are grains like quinoa, barley, and riced or mashed cauliflower. However, be careful not to add too much butter or oil. Try adding a variety of spices, including garlic and salt (but not too much), to make these substitutes tastier.

You must also eliminate all snack foods and desserts. Yes, I know that's hard to do, but two to three days after you kick the sugar addiction, you will be pleasantly surprised with yourself. Because your intake of fresh fruits and veggies is unlimited, snack on fruits, veggies, and a few nuts (e.g., almonds and cashews) instead. But be careful with nuts. The calories can really add up quickly. And peanuts are not allowed (they are actually legumes).

Although the Farmhouse Diet is not a low-fat diet per se, choose leaner cuts of meat. Use added fats and oils sparingly. Eggs are also allowed—and are actually good for you—but use only egg whites during Phase 1. Skim milk is rather nutritious and filling and can be used to make a satisfying shake or smoothie. However, no cheese is allowed in this phase.

It is important that you do not eat out during this phase. In fact, it is probably best to avoid any travel during Phase 1 because you may lose control of your diet while on the road. Have you ever thought about bringing your lunch to work or school? A novel idea in modern times, but try it.

There are two more rather austere aspects of the induction phase of the diet: no alcohol and no sweets. However, contrary to other popular diets, caffeine is not off-limits. The possible negative effects it may have on your weight loss are rather minor and not well substantiated. And what's better for you as a treat . . . a little espresso or cup of coffee with artificial sweetener and skim milk or a donut? If a fully caffeinated diet soda is what it takes to get you through the afternoon until your healthy supper, then go for it.

There are two really good ways to hold yourself accountable for your weight loss and healthy lifestyle. First, write down your goals for the week, such as losing two pounds, attending an online support group, drinking one homemade smoothie per day, cutting out sweet tea, or exercising for thirty minutes on Saturday, Sunday, and Wednesday. Second, keep a food diary. Yes, you really need to write down everything you eat, as well as the amount and the time of day that you eat it. You will also later need to add a notation about whether you were really hungry or not when you ate. Make a note of whether your hunger was satisfied or not. Look for patterns in when your hunger recurs and note if you experience symptoms of dumping syndrome. In medicine, we put great emphasis on collecting data. However, we must also analyze the data if we want to improve outcomes. The same applies to improving your weight and lifestyle. You can use a simple blank chart like the one that follows.

SAMPLE FOOD DIARY PAGE

	Monday	Tuesday	Wednesday	Thursday	Friday	Saturday	Sunday
Breakfast							
Snack							
Lunch							
Snack							
Dinner							

This Week's Goals: _____

_____

_____

_____

The second really good way to hold yourself accountable is to find a weight-loss and/or exercise partner to not only encourage you but also understand your struggles and exhort you to meet your goals.

Some people do better with a coach—for example, a personal trainer or nutritionist—holding them accountable, rather than a partner. These partners can be found at local weight-loss support groups. Also, church members or your neighbors may fit the bill. Avoid family members, however, because they can often be overly critical and sometimes sabotage you.

PHASE 1: EAT

Fresh fruit

Fresh vegetables

Protein shakes and no-added-sugar smoothies

Nuts (but not peanuts) sparingly

Lean meat, especially fish

Skim milk

Yogurt

Egg whites

Spices and seasonings

PHASE 1: DON'T EAT

Fried foods

Potatoes

Pasta

Rice

Bread

Cheese

Processed snack foods

Fast food

Sugary drinks

Phase 2: The Diet

You may not have enjoyed the first phase of the Farmhouse Diet, but you can celebrate your successful completion of it and your awesome weight loss! Now comes the really exciting and satisfying part of the diet, Phase 2, in which you will discover healthy and delicious foods that result not only in weight loss but also in feeling better. You will also feel better about yourself as you continue to meet your goals and improve health and fitness. And if you fall off the wagon, there is still hope. You can get back on it and continue to meet your goals.

The length of time you are on this phase of the diet depends on your weight-loss goal. Remember, you need to be realistic about how much weight you can expect to drop. Long-term maintenance of your weight and improved health are more important than hitting an ambitious weight-loss goal. A reasonable goal would be to lose one pound per week.

To maximize your success, make a commitment to learning to cook or learning new techniques. Not only is eating a meal that you created yourself rewarding, but it is also cheaper and healthier than the equivalent premade or restaurant food. If done right, it's also tastier. And it's great fun for the whole family!

In Phase 2, you can add whole-grain breads and whole-wheat pasta. A small amount of potatoes is OK, but consider potato substitutes, as listed in the next section. You can add some alcohol in moderation, but no more than two servings per week (a serving is 12 oz for beer and 4 oz for wine). Choose light beer over regular beer, and keep in mind that craft beers may have substantially more calories.

You can have an indulgence such as pizza (but not the whole pizza!) or a burger once per week, but remember that too much indulging will subvert your dieting efforts. You may have dessert once per week. However, two pieces of dark chocolate per day, 85 percent or more cacao, are also allowed. Because dark chocolate is mostly cacao and does not have much added sugar or many carbs, healthwise, it is superior to milk chocolate and almost all sweets. It is also full of antioxidants, a nutrient associated with better health. Make sure it does not contain added nuts. This, of course, excludes candy bars. Dried fruits are very high in calories, so avoid those as well, except as a special indulgence. Beware of ice cream. There is no such thing as diet ice cream.

Now that you've kicked your sugar addiction and no longer desire sugary drinks, be sure to drink plenty of water. People who formerly did not like the taste of water will now be refreshed by a cold drink of water.

When planning and serving meals, utilize the Farmhouse Plate. There are two different plates for you to choose from:

Option 1: 1/2 veggies, 1/4 proteins, 1/4 healthy carbs
(not potatoes, rice, pasta, or bread, except the
whole-grain varieties)

Option 2: 1/2 veggies, 1/3 proteins, 1/6 healthy carbs
(see Figure 4-1)

Notice that there is not a slice for dessert or sweet tea. That's because desserts and sweet drinks are not part of a meal. These are special treats. But you can eat all the fresh fruit that you desire! Dairy is also not its own slice because it may be included in the carb or protein slices, depending on carb and protein content. Some dishes may have components of multiple slices, like most casseroles.

Breakfast should consist of eggs, lean proteins, yogurt, and fresh fruits rather than the traditional *diaita Americana* breakfast of sugary

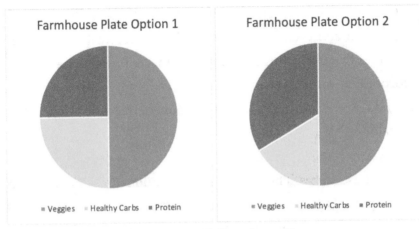

Figure 4-1. The Farmhouse Plate

cereals and pastries. Whole-grain cereals are OK but may not be optimal for weight loss. Use skim milk in cereals because it is lower in fat and calories than whole milk. If you are having a hard time finding palatable selections for breakfast, or if you're short on time, consider simply drinking a protein shake or smoothie for breakfast. I often drink 12 oz of V8 juice for breakfast.

Breakfast has been described as the most important meal of the day, but is it possible that it is the least important meal of the day? If skipping a meal makes you more ravenous and causes you to overindulge later, then do not skip a meal. Otherwise, consider continuing your overnight fast, consuming only sugar-free beverages until lunch. And of course, eat a healthy lunch. The jury is still out on whether skipping breakfast is helpful or detrimental.

Limit eating out to one lunch and one supper per week, and do not go to a buffet. Bring your lunch to work or school. Emphasize cooking at home. Also, fried foods, processed foods, packaged foods, and snack foods are still off-limits. This includes french fries, chips, crackers, and cookies.

Increase the amount of grains and fresh vegetables in your diet. Frozen and even canned vegetables are acceptable. However, vegetables in certain forms, such as from a Chinese restaurant or incorporated into a casserole (e.g., green bean casserole) are not much different from eating a pizza because of the added ingredients and calories.

Eat fish or seafood at least two or three times per week.

Don't use sauces. They can add a tremendous amount of calories and simple sugars. Add herbs and seasonings, as well as a little butter or olive oil. Use only light salad dressings, and avoid creamy dressings. Oil-based dressings are better. All salad dressings should be used in moderation. Toss the dressing into the salad well. If the dressing pools at the bottom of your bowl, you have used too much.

The list of substitutes in chapter 7, under "Basic Food-Prep Techniques," and the "eat/don't eat" list later in this chapter will help you make healthier choices and create delicious meals.

Be a smart consumer and dieter. Foods that are advertised as healthy may actually be nothing of the sort. For example, don't get fooled into thinking that wheat bread is healthy. It is just processed flour. Look for stone-ground whole-wheat bread instead. So-called healthy chips, such as lentil chips, may have potato starch listed as the first ingredient, with less than 10 percent of the chips made from lentils! Look at the first ingredient on the package. Is it flour, sugar, or potato starch? If so, then don't eat it.

Exercise remains a critical component of weight loss and fitness, as in Phase 1. See chapter 5 for more on exercise. You should continue to increase the amount of time you exercise and the degree of difficulty, such as running longer and faster. Exercise becomes easier and more enjoyable as weight drops and your cardiovascular stamina improves.

Continue your accountability with a diet and exercise partner, support group, or coach. Diet and exercise logs (see chapter 5 for an exercise log) will continue to be useful for meeting your goals. Write down your goals for the week, such as making healthy home-cooked meals every weeknight, bringing your lunch to work, eating a low-sugar grain cereal for breakfast, eating cooked whole grains instead of potatoes at supper, or driving right past the McDonald's. Weigh yourself two or three times per week. Don't forget that if you periodically fail, all hope is not lost. You can get back on track again!

PHASE 2: EAT

Whole-grain pasta

Whole-grain breads

Brown rice and whole grains

Potato substitutes

Fresh fruit

Fresh vegetables

Nuts (but not peanuts) sparingly

Lean meat, especially fish

Skim milk

Yogurt

Eggs

Cheese

Dark chocolate

PHASE 2: DON'T EAT

Fried foods

Processed snack foods

Fast food

Sauces

Casseroles

Sugary drinks

A PERSONAL JOURNEY

How I Lost Twenty-Five Pounds

The first two weeks of my diet were particularly austere. During that time, I ate zero bread, potatoes, fried food, pasta, and desserts. Within a couple of days, I realized I had a sugar addiction. It was tough, and I never really intended to keep that phase up, but I did lose five pounds in the first week!

After the first two weeks, I decreased sugar, decreased wheat, really decreased potatoes, decreased bread, decreased pasta, really decreased processed foods, really decreased desserts, eliminated sugary drinks and snacks, decreased fried food, practically eliminated fast food, decreased eating out, and cooked more at home. Take note that I only decreased intake and did not completely eliminate anything except sugary drinks and snacks.

I still ate any and all fruits, meats, nuts, and even some chocolate. I ate lots of salads and veggies. I did not go hungry. I did not watch fat intake, but I did avoid fried and greasy foods. I even had occasional wine and beer but in greater moderation.

Most of my meals were at home. And I'm by no means a gourmet cook, which proves that an average person with little culinary skill can still prepare delicious and healthy home-cooked meals. I did need to—and even desire to—eat out sometimes. I tried to go for the healthier options. But I also occasionally skipped a meal because there were no healthy options on the road.

Exercise was and still is a critical component. I typically run about fifteen to twenty miles per week.

I still ate my yummy whole-grain-based cereal, but with less sugar. Some days, I had V8 and a slice of bacon for breakfast! Usually, I broke the diet about once a week.

I've kept the weight off by maintaining those healthy lifestyle changes, weighing myself frequently, dieting, and eating lots of good food—including carbs, fats, meats, and some sweets. And if my weight creeps up, I'll diet again. I still usually try to keep my carbs to about one-fourth of my plate, and I still only rarely eat fast foods, snack foods, and processed foods. But I also have indulgences. In fact, as I sit here in the Embassy Suites in Memphis writing this, I plan on indulging in the manager's special tonight!

A year later, I'm still doing great. Although I failed over Christmastime and picked up a few pounds, I'm slowly taking that back off.

How My Wife Lost Twenty Pounds

She did it differently than I did and has been every bit as successful, which proves that there are many paths to successful dieting and lifestyle changes.

She did not decrease potatoes, starches, or fruit, nor did she eliminate fast food and prepackaged foods. She did increase exercise, reduce her total intake of calories, and decrease snacking and desserts.

Both of us have been successful, but we each took different approaches.

Confessions of a Sugar Addict

I did not know that I had a sugar addiction until I came off it! The first few days were rough, but then I felt much better and full of energy. Over Halloween and Christmas, my weight crept back up again. Guess why?

My Running Program

My best friend, an emergency medicine doctor in Wisconsin, challenged me to run a 10k with him when we were planning a trip to visit him and his family. I took up the challenge. But because I had stopped running years before and was basically an overweight couch potato, I knew I needed to train. So I spent ten weeks preparing. The first week was brutal. I could run only for about five minutes, then had to walk for about ten minutes. But after the first two weeks, I could run about three miles without stopping. I added about a mile per week until I could run over seven miles! Yes, I was fairly slow, but I could do it. The day of the big race, I had my best time ever and felt great.

After that success, I continued training. I developed a sensible program in which I ran three to four times per week, almost always in the morning, when I am at my best. Over the next two months, I was able to run about a mile farther every week on my "long run." I lost about seven pounds in the process without really dieting. This culminated in me running my first half marathon. That's 13.1 miles! From couch potato to athlete—if I could do it, so can you.

Since my first half marathon, I've lost twenty to twenty-five pounds and run two more half marathons and other races. In fact, I've substantially increased my speed and can run without getting winded. My knees no longer hurt when exercising, and my cardiovascular health has improved greatly. At fifty, I'm healthier now than I was in my thirties. I continue to exercise three or four mornings a week. There's no looking back.

Phase 3: Your New Lifestyle

You did it! You reached your weight-loss and fitness goals. Now is the phase when you will maintain your weight and level of fitness. This phase, your new lifestyle, is the rest of your life. So make sure that your goals and new diet habits are realistic.

Nothing is off-limits per se, regardless of the calorie count. As long as the food is fresh or cooked with very small amounts of added fat and sugar, you can eat it. Beware of canned and prepackaged fruits and veggies, added sugar, and vegetables cooked in a restaurant because they usually have a lot of added fat and even sugar.

Weigh yourself frequently, two or three times per week, at the same time of day and with the same amount of clothes on. Do it before you exercise or after, but be consistent so that you will get a true picture of your weight. It's not uncommon to lose a couple of pounds during an intense aerobic workout. Weighing weekly is probably not enough to hold yourself accountable, but weighing every day is probably counterproductive.

Continue to use the Farmhouse Plate. Continue to use healthy substitutes. Have a daily eating plan, such as eating sweets only twice per week, avoiding juices at breakfast, not going back for seconds, or never eating fried foods at lunch. Yes, it may sound a bit obsessive-compulsive to plan what you will eat every day a week in advance, but this will keep you from carelessly and insidiously packing on the pounds.

You may eat some processed and snack foods in this phase, but do it in moderation. Alcohol, desserts, and other indulgences should also be occasional; moderation is key. Be careful of what you eat on vacation and during the holidays, or be prepared to lose that extra five pounds when they're over!

Set a standard for yourself as to how often you will eat out at a restaurant and what kinds of foods you will allow yourself. You may want to continue to limit eating out to once or twice per week, unless you are traveling or have a business lunch. Set limits, such as indulging in either an appetizer or a dessert but not both. Limit yourself to one serving of alcohol, and order no more than one side item. Select a fish or seafood option one out of three times when eating out. If you eat pizza or a burger, make sure you also order a salad instead of eating fries or more pizza.

Stay committed to cooking and eating at home. Family meals are the cornerstone of the traditional American family. You should teach your new healthy lifestyle to others, including your spouse and children. The nuclear family can potentially be the best support system for your new healthy lifestyle, but they have to understand and buy into it.

Make goals each week, such as eating fish and vegetables at a restaurant rather than steak and fries, drinking one light beer when grilling pork tenderloin on Saturday, making your own broth-based soup, skipping the desserts at a church function, or running a 5k.

CHALLENGES

Make a diet plan.

Take your lunch to work.

Cook at home five nights per week.

Limit yourself to eating out twice per week.

Don't eat fast food.

Eat healthy when on business trips or vacation.

Skip dessert.

Don't skip breakfast if it makes you ravenous later in the morning.

Eat healthy snacks, such as fresh fruit, fresh veggies, and nuts (sparingly).

Be accountable, not only to yourself but also to another dieter.

Stick with those good eating and lifestyle changes that you made in Phase 2.

The hardest part of a diet is sticking to it. The aim of the Farmhouse Diet is to create a reasonable eating plan consistent with lifestyle changes for long-term success with weight control. Whether you're a longtime dieter, had weight-loss surgery or an intragastric balloon, have taken diet medications, or had no interventions at all, the Farmhouse Diet is a powerful tool for your continued success. In the long run, I never say no to anything. Moderation and identifying your diet struggles and addictions are the keys to success. Do you have a problem with carbs, fast food, or alcohol? Then those are areas you will need help with avoiding or moderating. Having someone who holds you accountable and avoiding situations that trigger your desire for problem foods are important.

Have a plan in the event of recidivism and weight regain. Go back to Phase 2 or even Phase 1. But whatever you do, don't give up. You can get the weight back off. It's not hopeless. You are not a failure.

Exercise is very important not only for losing weight but also for keeping it off. Make a goal, for example, of working out three hours per week in a gym, running fifteen miles per week, or walking three miles per day. At first, it will be very difficult, exhausting, and even demoralizing when starting a new exercise program. But don't feel like a failure. Keep at it, and you'll be surprised at what you can do. See chapter 5 for more on exercise.

PHASE 3: EAT

Meat

Dairy: butter (in moderation), milk, yogurt, and so
forth; no ice cream

Eggs

Fresh fruits and veggies

Whole-grain breads and pasta

Scottish or steel-cut oatmeal

Potatoes (in moderation)

Grains such as quinoa, barley, and millet

Beans and lentils

Soups with clear broth

Fish and seafood

Sautéed foods, particularly in extra-virgin olive oil

PHASE 3: DON'T EAT

So-called "nonfat" foods, which contain substantial
amounts of sugar

High-fat foods

Foods with added sugar

Foods containing high-fructose corn syrup

Processed foods

Canned fruit

Too much starch

Instant or Quaker-style oatmeal (which is mostly
simple carbs with a high glycemic index)

Grits

Only protein or meat instead of vegetables

Creamy soups

Fried foods

Fast food

FOODS THAT MAKE YOU HUNGRY AGAIN IN A COUPLE OF HOURS

Any snack food in a box

Pancakes and French toast

Candy

Sweets, pastries

Chinese food with monosodium glutamate (MSG)

Fruit juice and sugary smoothies

Low-fat yogurt

Granola bars

Sugary cereal

CHAPTER 5

Walk, Run, Race!

Another important facet of the Farmhouse Diet is exercise. Exercising will synergize with your dietary changes to improve your weight, health, and fitness. In general, you should exercise three or four times per week at the time of day when you have the most energy. This may be first thing in the morning or after work. Some people may go to the gym during their lunch break. Make an appointment to exercise, and don't break it. Put it on your calendar, or make a log of when you start and stop exercising. The Fitbit phenomenon and other health trackers, along with fitness apps, have made it easier than ever to track your exercise. They can even be used to push your performance and achieve goals. Consider finding a friend to exercise with you on certain days. With these apps, your exercise buddy does not even need to be in the same state you are in!

Obviously, your exercise schedule will have to be compatible with your work or school schedule. Sometimes, busy people can only find time to exercise on the weekends. If you cannot find regular time during the week to exercise, perhaps your leisure time on the weekends can revolve around outdoor and other physical activities. Busy moms may best exercise with other moms after dropping the kids off at school. If at the ball fields with the kids, plan on walking around the fence or on the track every time you are there. Better yet, coach them and get the extra exercise.

SAMPLE EXERCISE CALENDAR

Sunday:	Walk or run for one hour in the early morning
Monday:	Day off
Tuesday:	Day off
Wednesday:	Do cardio in the gym for one hour, either before work or after
Thursday:	Day off
Friday:	Go to the gym before or after work
Saturday:	Walk/run, or do a special exercise event, such as biking, hiking, running a race, or some strenuous outdoor family activity

If you enjoy running, for example, make one of your exercise goals to run a 5k or a half marathon or even compete in a triathlon.

Make time to exercise, and have alternate plans in the case of bad weather, travel, and illness. If you are used to running or walking, have a backup plan of riding an exercise

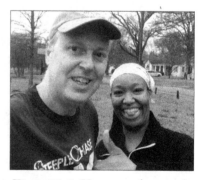

Figure 5-1. You never know who you'll meet exercising in the park!

bike, using a NordicTrack, or mall walking instead. Look for nearby jogging paths and fitness centers in the hotel whenever traveling.

When exercising, you need to get your heart rate up and sweat. It should be somewhat strenuous and tiring. The recommended intensity varies based on your general health and conditioning, as well as your fitness goals. For weight loss, it's important to do aerobic types of exercise, such as walking, running, cycling, and rowing, rather than nonaerobic exercise, such as strength training. Do not lift weights in this phase. Note that your weight may not change as much as you would expect, but your waist size will decrease as you build muscle with aerobic exercise. It would not be uncommon to put on ten pounds in muscle, yet lose even more in fat as your strength and endurance increase.

Standing for long periods of time and lots of walking at work do not count much as exercise. Standing for an hour only burns about nine more calories than sitting. Although you may be tired after doing certain chores, you may be surprised at how few calories common household activities actually burn, as shown in the following chart.

CALORIES BURNED						
Daily Activities	**175 lbs**	**200 lbs**	**225 lbs**	**250 lbs**	**275 lbs**	**300 lbs**
Cleaning the kitchen	90	102	114	128	141	153
Shopping	95	108	122	135	149	162
Cooking	105	120	135	150	165	180
Walking, moderate pace	146	167	188	208	229	250
Playing with children	158	180	203	225	248	270
Sex	168	192	216	240	264	288
Dancing	237	270	303	338	372	405
Aerobics	315	360	405	450	495	540
Calories burned over a 30-minute period by activity at a particular weight.						

Figure 5-2. Calorie expenditures for common daily activities

Keep a log of your exercise as well. If you run or walk, there are lots of apps for smartphones that will keep track of your mileage, time, and even calories burned. You can share the data with your friends to keep you motivated and celebrate your successes.

EXERCISE LOG					
Date	Activity	Time Spent	Avg. Heart Rate	Mileage	Calories Burned

Drink plenty of water before, during, and after exercise. There's no problem with taking a bathroom break during your exercise routine; just don't lose the momentum. You may want to avoid caffeine prior to exercising because this may send you to the bathroom more frequently!

Water aerobics and slow-paced swimming are good exercises, as are stretching and yoga, but they are not sufficient to burn enough calories to result in weight loss. To lose weight, you will need to increase your heart rate for around thirty minutes daily, but sixty minutes is better.

During exercise, you should raise your heart rate significantly higher than your resting rate to achieve maximal health and weight-loss benefits. To estimate your maximum heart rate, subtract your age from 220. Your target average heart rate for burning fat should be 70 percent of that number. For example, a fifty-year-old person should have a target heart rate of 120 beats per minute during exercise. A Fitbit or other fitness tracker is very useful for constantly monitoring your heart rate.

Formula: (220 – your age [years]) × .7 = your target heart rate

Don't be disappointed by terrible results when you first start exercising. You will fail. But be persistent, and you will ultimately win. Start by taking a daily walk. If the weather is inclement, walk in your local mall or a large office complex. The next step may be to join a gym and actually use the gym membership. "I have a gym membership" is not equal to "I exercise regularly."

If you want to be a runner, you will have to start with walking. Anticipate

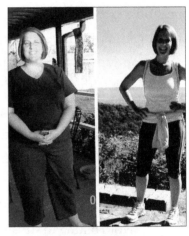

Figure 5-3. *Before and after diet and exercise*

that you will need to take lots of breaks. When you first start to run, you may only be able to run for five minutes, then slow down to a fast walk. Walk for five minutes, and then try to run for another five. After about a week of daily running/walking, you should be able to run for about fifteen minutes without stopping. After two weeks of daily running, set the goal of running three miles within forty-five minutes. After that, cut back to three or four days of running per week. Push your goals to become a bit faster and run a bit longer every week. If you get into the habit of running farther, you may need longer periods between runs. One, two, or even three days of rest may be necessary for your body to recover. This is not a running book, but hopefully, this will get you started.

Many people need a coach not only to help design an exercise plan but also to push them to achieve their goals. You may want to join a gym that provides trainers; these individuals can ensure you are using proper body mechanics, as well as other forms of support. Most quality gyms have a variety of equipment for both aerobic and anaerobic exercises. Try the rowing machine, the treadmill, and either an upright or recumbent exercise bike. An elliptical or stepper is also a great option. To avoid getting stuck in a boring rut, change it up periodically with different machines.

When determining which type of exercise for weight loss is best for you, a good rule of thumb is that if a particular part of the body hurts, do not exercise that part. If you have bad knees, bike or row instead of running or walking. If you have impaired balance or mobility, consider water aerobics or swimming. Some people may want to avoid biking for reasons obvious to them. But they definitely don't want to *sit* it out. Some folks may complain that they hurt all over! With as little as a ten- to fifteen-pound weight loss, those body pains may "mysteriously" go away.

For those with heart disease, balance problems, diabetes, or a history of stroke, consult your physician before beginning a new exercise routine to find out which types are safest for you. Do not start a new exercise routine with unresolved medical issues, such as uncontrolled diabetes or high

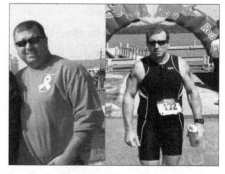

Figure 5-4. Couch potato to triathlete

blood pressure, heart disease requiring new medicines or interventions, or new symptoms such as dizziness or falling. Arthritis in the knees or hips, as well as low back pain, will require lower-impact exercises.

With this new commitment to exercise and fitness, don't be surprised if you put on ten pounds in muscle with aerobic exercises such as running. With weight-training exercises, you may gain even more muscle mass.

Consider joining an exercise class. Most fitness centers, YMCAs, and local communities have classes available for novices, older people, and those with a larger body habitus.

As with any good habit, including diet and a healthy lifestyle, developing an exercise routine takes hard work, dedication, and persistence. Also as with any good habit, you will reap the rewards of your labor.

EXERCISE TIPS

Exercise at the time of day that you perform best. Be consistent and start at about the same time on days that you exercise.

Set a progressive goal.

Make a schedule and stick to it as much as possible. Plan and look forward to your exercise the evening before.

Be flexible about how long and how vigorously you exercise.

Use opportunities to exercise, such as sprinting up the stairs, mowing the grass, and riding bikes with the family.

Don't have an all-or-nothing attitude. If you have less time to exercise than you expected, do it anyway. If your routine gets cut short, it still counts.

Keep a log of your exercise.

Get your heart rate up.

Drink plenty of water.

Choose an exercise routine that is a joy, not a chore.

Don't give up.

CHAPTER 6

A Trip to the Market

Even if you generally do not enjoy shopping, a trip to the grocery store can be fun and edifying. The market is full of exciting smells, shapes, and colors. It has its own special ambiance. In embracing the Farmhouse Diet, you get to select fresh meats, produce, grains, and spices; build a menu; learn new recipes; cook a masterful meal; eat your creation; nourish your family; and repeat. For the modern consumer, it all begins in the market.

To maximize your time and enjoyment, as well as to avoid sabotaging your diet, you will need to have a strategy when you go shopping. Otherwise, you may end up with junk food or processed food you never intended to buy in your grocery cart. If you come prepared, you will also avoid buying things that you do not need and wasting money. Do not make the mistake of wandering aimlessly around the aisles. Remember not to shop on an empty stomach. You'll end up buying more than you intended, especially low-nutritional-value foods.

Shop for fresh foods that you will cook and prepare at home. Avoid the aisles with a plethora of prepackaged, processed foods. Shopping at a farmer's market may be your best bet. It's much easier to find fresh foods than it was in the past. In recent years, there has been a movement back toward foods that are locally produced. Many are also organic and sustainable. Consider going to the market two or three times a week, or even daily, to keep your food fresh and tasty.

Come to the market with a grocery list. You will be less likely to buy things compulsively, including unhealthy foods that you do not need. Do not buy too much, or it may go to waste. And because of poor planning, you may end up just ordering a pizza instead.

Shop the periphery of the supermarket, where vegetables, meats, and dairy are located. Do not linger in the central part of the store, where processed foods and snack foods predominate. Make your first stop the produce section, then move on to the butcher shop and the seafoodmarket. Next, dairy. The bakery is often positioned near the entrance of the store, so skip it and come back at the end of your shopping experience.

Avoid foods that have more fat than protein. This includes any type of pork or beef sausage (turkey and chicken sausage are OK), hot dogs, bacon, bologna and salami, full-fat dairy (an exception is full-fat or Greek yogurt), peanuts, peanut butter, and almond butter. Seeds and nuts, if consumed in moderation, are allowed.

Rather than using oils and fats, sugar, and excess salt to season your foods, choose spices. There are many more spices and seasonings beyond salt and pepper, garlic and onion, and ketchup and mustard. For an exotic adventure, go to a specialty spice store. There are literally hundreds if not thousands of single spices and spice blends to add excitement to your dishes.

Nutrition Labels

The number of servings in a container or package, as well as the size of a serving, is prominently displayed at the top of the nutrition label.

This can be a bit deceptive, though, because the serving size does not always reflect the quantity that people actually eat. Most people eat more than the serving size. For example, the serving size on a can of Coke used to be labeled as 8 oz, but the can contains 12 oz. And while we're on that topic, who really eats three M&M's?

The calorie content in a serving is also prominently displayed. However, calorie counting is not as useful for your dieting efforts as carefully examining the fat, carbohydrate, and protein content.

Nutrition Facts
8 servings per container
Serving size 2/3 cup (55g)

Amount per serving
Calories 230

	% Daily Value*
Total Fat 8g	10%
Saturated Fat 1g	5%
Trans Fat 0g	
Cholesterol 0mg	0%
Sodium 160mg	7%
Total Carbohydrate 37g	13%
Dietary Fiber 4g	14%
Total Sugars 12g	
Includes 10g Added Sugars	20%
Protein 3g	
Vitamin D 2mcg	10%
Calcium 260mg	20%
Iron 8mg	45%
Potassium 240mg	6%

* The % Daily Value (DV) tells you how much a nutrient in a serving of food contributes to a daily diet. 2,000 calories a day is used for general nutrition advice.

(For educational purposes only. These labels do not meet the labeling requirements described in 21 CFR 101.9.)

***Figure 6-1.** Nutrition label*

The "% Daily Value" column tells you how much of that particular nutrient a serving of that food contributes to your daily dietary needs. It is based on the assumption of a diet of two thousand calories per day.

Note the breakdown of total fats, saturated fats, and trans fat. For weight loss and good health, avoid trans fats and saturated fats. The total grams of fat one eats per day is not as important as the type of fat and its source. A good rule of thumb is to choose proteins first, then fats, then carbohydrates.

Also note that carbohydrates are broken down by total as well as fiber and added sugar content. Keep sugar less than 15 g per serving. Do your best to limit yourself to 25 g of added sugar per day. Even less is better for actively losing weight. Of course, naturally occurring sugars in foods do not count toward your daily limit. The higher the fiber content of a food, the healthier it is.

The label also highlights total protein. Quality proteins have 8 g of protein per 100 calories. Most people need at least 60 g of protein per day, more if you are a larger person or trying to build muscle. During active weight loss in Phases 1 and 2 of the Farmhouse Diet, you may want to double your daily amount of protein.

Not all vitamins, minerals, and trace elements are listed, but they are all important. If you eat a healthy, varied diet, such as the Farmhouse Diet, then you should be meeting your daily requirements for vitamins, minerals, and trace elements. See chapter 2 for more information on vitamin supplements.

As mentioned earlier, come prepared by bringing a list to the store. A sample list follows.

Shopping List

Vegetable suggestions

Artichoke

Asparagus

Bean sprouts

Beets

Broccoli

Brussel sprouts

Cabbage

Carrots, including purple and white varieties

Cauliflower

Cucumbers

Eggplant

Green beans of various shapes and colors

Greens, including turnip, kale, Swiss chard, mustard, and collard

Lettuce, including bibb, romaine, iceberg, and so forth

Mushrooms

Okra

Onions

Peas

Peppers

Radishes

Rutabaga

Spinach

Squash

Tomatoes, including heritage varieties

Turnips

Zucchini

Protein suggestions

Beans of any kind (Note that they also contain starch and will have less total protein than meats.)

Chicken (Breast and wing are leaner than thigh and leg.)

Turkey (Breast is almost 100 percent protein.)

Avoid duck and goose, which are very fatty.

Beef (Select the leanest ground beef [93 percent lean, which still should be used sparingly] or lean steaks such as filet mignon, tenderloin, and top sirloin. Most other cuts, including pot roast, are fatty.) Bison can be very lean.

Wild game, such as deer (venison) and pheasant.

Pork loin (lean) and Canadian bacon

Fish, any kind, including the fattier salmon and tuna

Shellfish, such as shrimp, crab, and lobster

Eggs

Low-fat cheese

Cottage cheese

Tofu

Starch or carb suggestions

Sweet potato or yams

Butternut, spaghetti, and acorn squash

Steel-cut oatmeal

Whole-grain and multigrain breads

Brown rice

Quinoa

Bulgur wheat

Buckwheat

Kasha

Beans

Peas

Corn on the cob

Fruit, any kind, fresh (Avoid canned or cooked. Avoid pineapple, which is very sugary.)

Low-fat milk

Low-sugar yogurt

Foods high in fiber

Almost all fruits, including bananas, pears, oranges, apples, mangoes, strawberries, and raspberries

Beans

Legumes

Carrots, cauliflower, broccoli, brussels sprouts, green peas, turnip greens, and almost any dark-colored vegetable

Brown rice, whole-wheat spaghetti, oatmeal, quinoa

Grains, bran flakes, high-fiber cereals

Popcorn, almonds, sunflower seeds, pistachios

Some, but not all, whole-grain and multigrain breads

Notice that lettuce is not on this list!

The Spice Aisle

Smoked paprika, rosemary, dill, mint, cinnamon, chilies . . . are your taste buds tantalized yet? You *can* season with spices instead of fat and sugar. Basic seasonings such as garlic, salt, black pepper, oregano, and other spices can turn a healthy but somewhat bland dish into an exciting gourmet meal bursting with flavor. For the adventuresome epicurean gourmet, more "exotic" spices, like Chinese five-spice blend, cumin, cilantro, specialty salts, basil, tamarind, fennel, and curry powders bring true delight to one's dinner table. Dried mushrooms, although not actually a spice, can also add earthy flavors to a dish. Most seasonings, including the ones listed in this chapter, add no calories, nor do they have untoward health effects.

Blends of spices are used to create barbecues, vegetable medleys, and curries. Seasonings are used not only for meats but also for vegetables. The Savory Spice Shop in Franklin, Tennessee, is one of my favorite stores in the whole wide world. There are literally hundreds of choices of basic spices and seasonings as well as specialty blends.

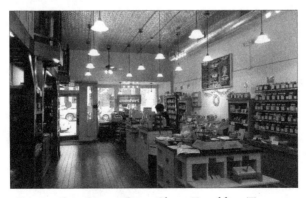

Figure 6-2. *Savory Spice Shop, Franklin, Tennessee*

List of Spices for Your Cabinet

Salt

Various specialty salts, like Himalayan pink salt, black salt, or sea salt

Salt-spice blends

Black pepper, white pepper, red pepper

Paprika

Ginger

Mint

Chili

Cinnamon

Dill

Star anise

Cardamom

Clove

Smoke flavoring

Bay leaves

Nutmeg

Lemon

Allspice

Peppermint

Vanilla

Cumin

Basil

Tamarind

Garlic

Fennel

Tarragon

Caraway seed

Turmeric

Coriander

Cilantro

Thyme

Oregano

Rosemary

Honey (sparingly)

Saffron

Mace

Poppy seed

Sorrel

For those of you who are still a little timid in the kitchen, partially and fully prepared meal kits are widely available in most areas of the country, either by mail, through delivery, or for pickup. Some kits are ready-made salads, casseroles, and healthier dishes that require reheating only. Others come with the raw ingredients and instructions on how to prepare the meal. Make it a goal to be able to follow a recipe without the aid of a meal kit. Using spice blends from the grocery store or specialty spice store on meats and veggies can help you create incredibly tasty meals without depending on prepackaged kits.

HelloFresh, Blue Apron, and Amazon Fresh are well-known food deliverers, but your local grocery store or other local company may provide a similar service. Be prepared to pay top dollar for the convenience.

Before you head out to the market, keep in mind what you want to buy that's consistent with your new diet and lifestyle, as well as what you *don't* want to buy.

BUY

Seasoning
Chicken or turkey sausages
Lean beef
Pork loin
Chicken
Fresh seafood
93 percent lean ground beef
Eggs
Milk
Cheese (real cheese)
Whole grains
Whole-grain breads
Fresh fruit
Fresh veggies
Beans
Olive oil

DON'T BUY

Sauces
Frozen casseroles
Beef or pork sausages
Canned soups
Frozen pizza
French fries
Chips
Margarine
Processed or American cheese
White bread
Pastries
Anything in a box (except rice, whole-grain pasta, or grains)

CHAPTER 7

Cook. Serve. Eat. Repeat.

Can you boil water? Then you can cook!

Cooking is also a fun activity for the family. Involve the children, even the teens. Participation is a great way to introduce the family to healthy at-home cooking and eating. Young children love to be involved with cooking and following recipes.

Another family activity involving food would be to plant a garden and eat its produce. This can be done even in an urban setting. Can you imagine having farm-to-table in your own household?

Cooking Tips

Add:

> Spices and seasonings
>
> Salt (reasonable amounts)
>
> Fat-free broth or stock
>
> Oil, especially olive oil (pour into your own spritzer, potentially using less total oil)
>
> Butter (sparingly)
>
> Milk (skim or 1 percent)
>
> Garlic and onions
>
> Veggies

Don't add:

Too much salt

Too much oil

Margarine

Cream or creamer

Coconut milk

Sauces from a can or jar

Grilling Tips

Go low fat. (Add a small amount of uncooked bacon to the lowest-fat ground beef or bison for some extra flavor in your burger.)

Use lean beef, pork, venison, and chicken.

For better flavor, don't grill previously frozen meats.

It's not that hard to grill fish and shrimp, especially if you use a grilling basket.

Grill vegetables and fruits. (I grilled charred romaine last night, and, yes, you can grill even fruits!)

ANOTHER PERSONAL STORY

As a guy, I really enjoy grilling. Whole chickens, lean steaks, chicken, sausages, salmon, and pork tenderloin are some of my favorites. But I need to have a beer when grilling on the barbecue. It's a scientific fact that charred meat induces a craving for alcohol. However, after losing so much weight, I've redeveloped a little bit of a beer gut. Now it's time for low-carb beers. Because I can't stop grilling . . .

I also really enjoy hiking in the mountains. And what's better than a day of hiking followed by a visit to a craft brewery? Well, I figure that with all the calories burned on the hike, a couple of beers can be justified.

Basic Food-Prep Techniques

- Keep it simple.
- Use veggies in unexpected places, such as adding carrots to spaghetti sauce.
- Make healthy substitutions, such as sliced jicama with hummus or guacamole rather than pita or chips; sweet potatoes and other root vegetables for potatoes; mashed cauliflower for mashed potatoes; or grains such as quinoa, barley, buckwheat, and kasha for potatoes, rice, or pasta.
- Instead of pasta, use spaghetti squash or make "noodles" from zucchini using a spiralizer.
- Keep sliced and/or peeled fruits such as apples in a container in the fridge for snacking.
- For freshness, prep sliced melons or citrus fruit daily and keep them in the fridge for easy snacking access.
- Make whole-grain substitutions in foods such as pasta and breads.
- Add spices rather than excessive butter, cream, and sugar.
- Use herbs, and even vegetables, from your own garden. It always tastes better and is more satisfying if you grew it yourself!
- After cooking in a pan, drain out the grease.
- Avoid cream or sauces in making soups. Add pureed cashews or almonds to make them creamy.
- Use beef, chicken, turkey, fish, or vegetable broth (low fat) to add moisture and flavor to foods, especially when cooking rice and other grains.
- Steam, bake, or grill instead of frying. An air fryer is a good solution for low- or no-fat cooking.

- For baking, use almond flour, coconut flour, or whole grains instead of white processed flour.
- Avoid too much char on grilled meat. Char and overcooking can ruin the flavor, and charring is also thought to be unhealthy.
- To maximize flavor, don't overcook meats or veggies. Otherwise, you may have to add some sauce to make them palatable.
- Have fun!

Recipes

The Farmhouse Diet is not intended to be a cookbook, but a few tasty recipe ideas follow. Look up the details of these recipes in cookbooks or online. I hope you will be inspired to make some creations of your own.

Spaghetti squash with homemade marinara sauce

Zucchini "spaghetti" with garlic and olive oil and meatballs made from lean beef and turkey

Turkey stroganoff with spaghetti squash or spiralized zucchini

Cabbage tacos with fresh chicken, shrimp, or fish

Lettuce wraps with deli meat and avocado

Sesame carrot salad

Chinese salad with napa cabbage

Several types of soups

Borscht

Italian wedding soup

Lemon chicken quinoa soup

Vegetarian chili

Leftover Thanksgiving turkey white chili

Kale, potato, and turkey sausage soup

Spring vegetable soup

Creamy tomato basil soup made from pureed cashews

Pureed cashew and chestnut soup

Roasted vegetable medley (eggplant, mushrooms, cherry tomatoes, etc.)

Roasted chicken

Baked parmesan zucchini fries

Chicken stir-fry

Mashed or riced cauliflower

Baked sesame tofu

Chickpea burgers

Bison burgers

Jackfruit "pulled pork" barbecue

Protein bowl with farro wheat and avocado

Egg-white omelet with spinach, veggies, and Canadian bacon

White fish and cauliflower curry

Cioppino

Baked sweet potatoes with turkey chili or curried beans and lentils

Turkey sausage zucchini boats

Crab-and-shrimp-stuffed portobello mushrooms

Roasted, sauceless chicken wings with various seasonings

Shish kebabs with tenderloin, chicken, peppers, zucchini, and tomato

Potato-less ground turkey shepherd's pie

Spiralized zucchini "noodles" with pesto sauce

Greek shrimp-stuffed banana peppers

Bell peppers stuffed with ground tenderloin

Cauliflower-crust margherita pizza

Chicken salad made with roasted chicken breast and Greek yogurt, served on quinoa and brown-rice crackers

Italian tuna salad on sliced cucumber and jicama

Healthy Snack Suggestions

Carrots or celery and hummus

Cucumber and bell pepper with yogurt-based ranch dip

Anything with yogurt-based green goddess dip

Beef or turkey jerky

Guacamole with sliced jicama

Dark chocolate (85 percent or more cacao) with or without almonds

Nonbuttered popcorn

Sliced or peeled fruit or cherries and grapes

Sliced melon, including honeydew, cantaloupe, and watermelon

Rolled-up lunch meat

Low-fat cheese, like mozzarella or Babybel Light

Half-and-half mixture of cottage cheese and fresh fruit

Edamame, boiled and salted or dry roasted

Greek yogurt

Hardboiled egg with salt and pepper

Baked apple (no added sugar)

Faux banana ice cream made with pureed frozen bananas and skim or almond milk

Chia-seed protein pudding

Blueberry-lemon breakfast quinoa

include weight loss, a healthy diet such as the Farmhouse Diet, and specific medications for IBS.

Acid Reflux

Hopefully, with diet changes and weight loss, acid reflux will resolve. When substituting spices for fat and sugar, certain seasonings, especially hot or peppery spices, could make reflux worse. If symptoms persist, you may take an over-the-counter acid reducer like omeprazole. Tums and Rolaids are OK, too, but you should let your physician know about your symptoms. These medications could possibly mask an ulcer, gastritis, or esophagitis.

Dumping Syndrome

Dumping syndrome occurs when you eat something high in simple sugars or simple carbs. Symptoms include shakes, nausea, sweats, dizziness, weakness, and just feeling downright bad. Simple sugars and carbs are absorbed too quickly, causing your blood sugar to spike too quickly. This causes insulin to peak too early, which then, paradoxically, results in lowering your blood sugar too much. This is what people are experiencing when they complain of "low blood sugar." How do you avoid it? Don't eat foods with sugar or simple carbs. Go for complex carbohydrates.

Caffeine

Many physicians and dietitians advise their patients to stay off caffeine because they believe that caffeine will inhibit the patients' weight loss. However, there is no solid scientific evidence of that, and the effect would be modest anyway. Weight-loss diets make a lot of things off-limits, but you can indulge in at least one thing: caffeine—so enjoy that organic low-fat milk latte!

Artificial Sweeteners

Are artificial sweeteners bad for your health, and do they cause weight regain? That's a tough question to answer. There can be side effects of artificial sweeteners (even "natural" ones like stevia), such as bloating, gas, and even more cravings for sweets. For many artificial sweeteners, the long-term effects on health are unknown. My stance is that if you need an artificial sweetener to keep you from excess sugar, carb, and calorie intake, then it is fine to use it.

Special Note after Weight-Loss Surgery

Certain foods are challenging after having weight-loss, or bariatric, surgery. Dry or chewy meats and stringy vegetables are harder to digest. Fibrous foods, such as asparagus and celery, are harder to digest. Poultry (e.g., chicken breast or turkey), pork, and some tougher beef cuts are notoriously dry. Pasta, rice, and bread (unless toasted) don't pass out of your sleeve or pouch very quickly. "Slider foods," such as processed foods and those with excessive simple carbs and sugars, may pass through easily, but they are usually bad for your weight. They can also cause dumping syndrome, especially after a gastric bypass. Surprisingly, salads are easy to digest after about a month out from your weight-loss surgery.

Fatty, oily, greasy, or fried foods commonly cause diarrhea. This includes salad dressings, as well as veggies to which too much oil or butter has been added.

CHAPTER 9

Teen Weight Loss

Teen obesity in the United States has reached epidemic proportions. The current generation of young people may be the first ever for whom life span will decrease relative to that of previous generations. And it is all driven by obesity.

Clearly, the most important way to combat obesity in teenagers, who will, of course, later become adults and the elderly, is through the prevention of obesity in children. However, how do you intervene with adolescents who are already overweight or obese? The primary emphasis should be on healthy eating, healthy lifestyle changes, and activity. The same basic principles for adults also apply to teens. I encourage teens to read the entire book, not just this chapter.

Eating good food requires extra work and planning. It's easy to grab a poor-quality snack or fast food and much harder to plan and prepare a good-quality, nutritious meal. Food preparation, as well as doing meaningful exercise, requires a time commitment and thoughtful planning. These are adult skills and require training and parental assistance to execute.

It is important for teens to achieve a healthy weight. The passive expectation that your kid will just "grow out of it" is unlikely to be successful. There is much more danger from the comorbidities of obesity as a teen, and later as an adult, than from the potentially deleterious effects of reducing calories in a developing body.

There are other considerations for good nutrition in growing, changing bodies. Exercise and calcium are important to build bone strength in adolescents. Although a nutritious, varied diet should provide all the vitamins, calcium, and other minerals that a growing teen needs, consideration should be given to extra multivitamin and calcium supplementation. It almost certainly won't hurt. Menstruating girls may also need iron supplementation.

Another benefit of healthy eating is that avoiding simple sugars and simple carbs can go a long way in resolving acne in adolescents. In other words, do not eat junk food, and your skin will clear up. Everyone knows that sugary junk food causes dental caries, but did you know that soda (even diet soda) will weaken and erode teeth? Vitamin A, found in vegetables, eggs, nuts, and fish, is important for vision. Vitamin D, which is found in dairy, fish, eggs, and mushrooms, is important for strong bones.

It is an understatement to say that adolescent boys and girls undergo a lot of hormonal and body changes. With an increase in testosterone, boys can put on considerable muscle. Girls will have new deposits of fat on their hips, buttocks, and breasts. With the onset of menses, girls need iron to prevent anemia. Teens need extra calories and protein to develop properly. Healthy sources of proteins and calories, not low-density junk food, are important for proper development. Unhealthy food sources will lead to obesity.

Moms, I know that you are the ones reading this chapter and not your kids. So use this chapter, even this entire book, as a tool to graciously encourage your teen toward healthy eating, healthy exercise habits, and a healthy weight. Don't use it as a cudgel to hit them over the head. Encourage rather than punish. Pick one goal a week to work on, such as avoiding unhealthy snacks after school. Your teen needs to buy into the Farmhouse Diet to achieve long-lasting success with a healthy lifestyle. I will never forget my patient who was strong-armed by her mom into getting a Lap-Band as a teenager but rebelled and actually gained weight. Only years later, as an adult in her midtwenties, did she decide to take control of her weight and lifestyle. Building a healthy lifestyle takes time. The battles are won incrementally in small steps, not a big destructive battle. But it's so worth it.

TIPS FOR HEALTHY EATING AND LIFESTYLE CHANGES THAT YOUR HIGH SCHOOL OR COLLEGE TEEN CAN STICK TO

Bring lunch to school. Yes, I know that's not cool, but neither is being the fat kid.

Avoid eating out with friends after school.

Avoid gorging on food after school.

Eat a healthy breakfast. Repeat, eat breakfast!

Have fruit for a snack or no snack at all.

Avoid sugary drinks. For those raised on juice boxes and soda, this can be very difficult. Drink water instead.

With better nutrition, teens will find that they concentrate better, study better, and perform better in class. Healthy food in one's system is better than food that causes one's blood sugar to drop too rapidly.

Physical exercise in the form of walking to class, sports, or regular exercise is also important for achieving a healthy weight. Commitment to regular exercise may be difficult but is necessary.

For college kids living in a dorm, choose one with a well-equipped communal kitchen. Preparing a meal with friends is not only fun but also may be seen as a little offbeat (and therefore, now trendy).

Cafeteria food may sabotage weight-loss efforts. Cafeteria food is often high in simple carbs, low in quality protein, and full of sugar. When I was in high school, the teachers got a salad bar, the "rich" kids could eat from the burger and pizza line, and the rest of us were stuck with the mystery meat served up by the lunch lady. Oh, and ketchup was considered a vegetable. At many schools, healthy options are now available, but, sadly, many are stuck in the past.

CHAPTER 10

Nutrition for Life

So you've done the hard work and lost the weight—great job! Long term, you will be staying in Phase 3 of the Farmhouse Diet, your new lifestyle. To maintain your newfound health and healthy weight, you need to be aware of several things that could sabotage your success. You will also need to have a strategy for getting back on track if you experience weight regain or backslide into old habits. Eating out, traveling, indulging in the occasional sweet, and drinking alcohol are not necessarily bad if you know how to manage these things.

Frenemies

There will always be people who envy your success, who do not like your new lifestyle, or who do not want to accommodate your new eating habits. Frenemies may be coworkers, close friends, or even a spouse. Sometimes the motivation for their attitude is the concern that you are not eating enough; that limiting processed foods and fast foods is somehow a cruel, self-inflicted punishment; or that you are wasting away. These attitudes are ingrained in American society and will take work to change.

The best way to deal with frenemies is to educate them on the advantages of the Farmhouse Diet. Convince them not only that it is the healthiest diet but also that it worked for you and will work for them.

> ## PERSONAL HABITS TO ENCOURAGE A HEALTHY WEIGHT
>
> Get enough sleep.
>
> Rise early.
>
> Read or meditate.
>
> Stretch.
>
> Adhere to the Farmhouse Diet.

Alcohol

Fermented beverages (i.e., alcohol) have been a part of human culture for millennia. Regardless of your belief whether it's right or wrong to imbibe intoxicating drinks in twenty-first-century America, it is being done and will continue to be done well into the future. Prohibition proved that. Ancient texts, including the Bible, describe the fruit of the vine and grain beverages that produce joy. These glorious liquids were not only associated with celebration but also aroused the temptation to be abused. So the question at hand for us is this: Is there a place for alcohol for the serious dieter?

This book does not seek to answer the question of whether there are any health benefits of alcohol. Throughout history, it has been used medicinally but has also caused great destruction to individual bodies as well as whole societies. So for the serious dieter and the health-conscious individual, is alcohol permissible? The answer is yes.

Certainly, in the induction phase of your diet, it's important to avoid simple sugars and carbs. Eliminate all empty calories. This includes alcohol. Beer, especially craft beer, has a high calorie content. Ever wonder where a beer belly comes from? This is due to beer's high carb and sugar content. Most beer is wheat beer, but brewers utilize other grains as well. Fortunately, there are lower-calorie, lower-carb beers available with better taste and more variety than ever before. Wines are fruit based, usually grape, and have three times fewer carbs than regular beer. The drier wines are, in theory, less detrimental to your dieting efforts than sweet wines. Liquors such as gin, vodka, and whiskey have less sugar and fewer calories and carbs (zero carbs, in fact) per serving than beer and wine. Beware of cocktails, though, because they are likely to have quite a bit of added sugar. Just say no to the margarita or hurricane! Liquor with seltzer is less bad for you than alcohol with fruit-flavored or sweet mixes.

In summary, alcohol is OK for the serious dieter and the health-conscious individual, but it must be imbibed in moderation. It's certainly easy to overindulge. During the phase of most rapid weight loss (Phase 1), avoid alcohol. In subsequent phases, carefully limit alcohol intake by proscribing yourself limits and sticking to them—for example, one glass of red wine or two low-calorie/low-carb beers on the weekend. Or if you're at a social event or cocktail party, have only one serving of liquor mixed with seltzer, not a mixed drink. The limits you set for drinks are similar to those for the food you eat; aim for restraint and moderation.

Strategies for Vacations and Business Trips

You're on a business trip. Suddenly, you are out of your routine. Temptation abounds. It seems that the only food choices are bad ones.

There are strategies that you can employ to avoid blowing your weight goals. First, do not be afraid of missing out or losing money for not taking advantage of the free meals and snacks that may come with a hotel stay or that are supplied at a conference. These foods tend to be mostly low-nutritional-value processed foods, especially pastries.

Don't partake of that free hotel breakfast. People tend to eat about three times more than they would normally eat for breakfast at these big buffets. Waffles, bacon, sausage, bagels, pastries . . . these are typical offerings. Did I see some fruit hiding somewhere between the waffle maker and the pastries? It would be best to select yogurt, fresh (not canned) fruit, eggs, and some leaner meat. Consider that the best way to stick to your diet may be to bring your own protein shake on the trip and avoid the breakfast line.

Many hotels and conference centers offer evening specials and snacks between sessions. These are typically just bread, chips, and candy. Obviously, avoid these and choose veggies and lean meats instead. Hummus, guacamole, and salsa may be fine, but because you did not make them, you will not know what the added ingredients are. Alcohol can be a pitfall when traveling as well; follow the recommendations described earlier in this chapter.

When eating out on the road, select meat and veggies for a meal rather than potato, rice, and pasta options. Many restaurants now have calorie counts and healthier options on their menus. The caloric contents on the menu are often shocking. Rather than drinking soda, sweet tea, or alcohol, choose water. If eating soup, avoid creamy ones. Beware of salad dressings and toppings. Often, salads are not the healthiest items on the menu. Do not eat dessert. And of course, avoid fast food. Have a shake, protein bar, or fruit with you in the car. For a day trip, bring your lunch with you. Sometimes the only food choices on the road are bad ones, so it's best to be prepared.

When on a longer trip, consider staying in a suite with a kitchen. Taking a trip to a local market, shopping for fresh ingredients, and preparing a meal yourself in a new environment may actually be fun! Of course, the meal will need to be easy to prepare because you will have limited time and a very limited kitchen. You may need to make use of some prepackaged or premade foods.

When you are on vacation or even a business trip, make sure that you get in some time for exercise. Whether it's utilizing the hotel's gym or finding an exciting running route in a city that is new to you, it will be worth the extra effort in terms of both the health benefits and maximizing your travel pleasure.

When on vacation, it's not uncommon to pick up a few pounds. In fact, the typical person who takes a cruise gains one pound per day! With the strategies presented in this chapter, one can avoid weight gain and even lose weight.

After your trip, rather than wallowing in the guilt of having blown your diet, do a "Shake Your Boost" (see box later in this chapter), or put yourself in the recidivism program (see the following box and the section on recidivism that follows).

MY JOURNEY (BACK)

After great weight-loss success, I regained ten pounds over time. Vacations with big breakfasts, the "manager's special," and the Christmas holiday were my downfall. What a disaster! But all was not lost. I recommitted, and here's how I took off the extra ten pounds:

For breakfast, I had a protein bar and a V8 drink.

For lunch, I had a protein shake.

For dinner, I chose a healthy, high-protein, low-carb option—very filling, no limits on volume or calories.

I eliminated sweet drinks and desserts. (Well, I did have an occasional dark chocolate.)

I ate out only once or twice. This was at a steak house, where I had a lean filet, salad, and asparagus. I skipped the bread and potatoes.

I continued to exercise the entire time. I had no lack of energy because I was eating well and eating plenty.

At the end of twelve days, I started back on a sensible diet using the Farmhouse Diet principles found in this chapter and chapter 4. I made a commitment to watching my intake of simple carbs and sugar, as well as snack foods. Most importantly, I now have a plan to get back on track should I regain some weight in the future.

Recidivism: What to Do to Get Back on Track When You Have Regained Weight

It's normal to lose your focus on a healthy diet and lifestyle and backslide a bit. The question then becomes one of how to respond to weight regain and how to break out of old habits. Be encouraged, not discouraged! Focus on overcoming failure, focus on future success, and do not perseverate on past failures. Focus on pulling yourself up, overcoming your depression, and carrying on. Ignoring weight regain or a loss in fitness, becoming dejected and succumbing to hopelessness, and despairing that one is destined to become a fat slob is certainly a recipe for failure. But you can get back on track.

SHAKE THAT BOOST

If you've picked up a few pounds, which we all will do sooner or later, do not despair. Here is a strategy to get back to your fighting weight.

Basically, you will go back to the induction phase (Phase 1) of the Farmhouse Diet, adding in the optional two weeks of protein shakes in which you substitute protein drinks for some meals. Protein shakes should be high protein, low carb, and low sugar (not more than 1 g, but 0 g is preferred). You can make the protein shake yourself from a powder or drink a prepared shake.

Do at least two meals a day this way—all three if you have the willpower. If you are struggling to maintain an all-liquid protein-shake diet, then one meal could be a healthy meal of solid food that still fits the Phase 1 criteria. Also, you may be fighting to break the sugar addiction again, so the first five days of "Shake That Boost" could be rough.

After two weeks of protein shakes, if you have not already added back one healthy meal per day, do so now. After four weeks, resume Phase 3, your healthy lifestyle diet. (If you are achieving your goals, you can skip Phase 2.)

Adding a daily over-the-counter vitamin B12 supplement can be useful for boosting your energy. Also, have your physician check for other vitamin deficiencies. People with a vitamin D deficiency are often tired. Most middle-aged and older Americans should take a daily multivitamin as well.

Reclaiming Your Goal Weight and Fitness

Step 1. Admit that there is a problem and that you have failed.

Step 2. Redefine your goals. Was your original goal in terms of weight and fitness reasonable, attainable, and sustainable? Consider modifying your original goal. Ask yourself what it would really take to make you feel healthy and feel good about yourself. It is possible that you may have been too hard on yourself, too strict. If so, make new goals.

Step 3. Come up with a plan to achieve your goals. Select a healthy weight and a reasonable level of fitness for *you*. Consult a physician to help you find the right answer. Select a lifelong diet that you can actually adhere to.

Step 4. Set a start date for the induction phase, even if it means changing some of your plans and making some sacrifices. Use the "Shake That Boost" strategy. Make a realistic exercise schedule for three or more days a week. Put your exercise dates on the calendar. At the end of the week, assess your weight loss, change in pants size, number of minutes you can exercise vigorously, and so forth.

Step 5. Make a plan for when you fail (again). If and when that happens, get a coach. Go back to step 1. And plow through it.

The Seven Habits of Highly Effective Dieting

1. Fresh fruits and veggies.
   a. Avoid processed or canned vegetables and casseroles.
   b. You can have unlimited quantities; don't worry about calories.
   c. Nuts and seeds are not considered fresh fruits or veggies.
2. No fried, greasy, or oily foods.
   a. Chips, fries, fried chicken and fish, fried burgers, doughnuts, and so forth are off-limits.
   b. Watch oily and high-fat salad dressings.
3. No processed foods.
   a. No snack foods.
   b. No TV dinners, microwave meals, and so forth.

4. Whole grains and complex carbs are good.

    a. Avoid simple sugars and simple carbs, such as anything with potatoes, cornmeal or corn sugar, or added sugar. That includes sweets and desserts.

    b. Choose whole-grain pasta.

    c. Carefully select stone-ground whole-wheat breads.

    d. Choose grains such as buckwheat, barley, quinoa, and so forth.

5. Dairy, cheese, and eggs are good for you.

    a. Yes, you can eat an egg.

    b. Watch the fat content in cheese and milk.

    c. Full-fat yogurt is good for you.

    d. There's no such thing as diet ice cream.

6. Fats are OK.

    a. Make sure fat is not the foundation of your diet, however.

    b. Lean meats are generally better, but you can have beef, pork, chicken, and fish.

    c. Certain oils, like extra-virgin olive oil, are healthier than others.

7. Occasional "naughty" treats are OK.

    a. Avoid sugary beverages because they can contribute quite a few empty calories to your diet.

    b. Occasional desserts are OK, but they should be a treat, not a part of every meal.

    c. Alcohol, including beer and wine, is OK . . . again, in moderation.

    d. You can have bread with a meal. Just don't make it the whole meal.

Strategies for Dieting Success

1. Eat and cook at home.

    a. Avoid eating out. Most restaurants have very limited healthy options.

    b. Foods at restaurants almost always have much higher fat, carb, sugar, salt, and calorie counts than the equivalent food that you would cook at home.

    c. Don't know how to cook? Give it a try—it's actually fun!

2. Don't keep the "bad stuff" in the house.

    a. Even though it may be there for the kids, I guarantee that eventually you'll get into it.

    b. Keep fresh fruit sitting out on the counter to snack on instead of the bad stuff.

3. Keep engaged, active, and busy.

    a. Boredom leads to mindless snacking.

4. Read nutritional labels.

    a. The packaging and ads can be deceptive.

5. Artificial sweeteners are OK if they aid in compliance and reduce cheating.

    a. There are often gastrointestinal side effects of artificial sweeteners.

    b. The use of artificial sweeteners may prevent you from kicking your sugar addiction.

6. Stop eating when you start to feel full.

    a. Many people have the habit of stuffing themselves, especially during holidays.

7. You don't have to buy more expensive "organic" or gluten-free foods.

   a. Eating healthier can be more expensive, but you don't have to shop at an expensive specialty store to get healthy food.

   b. You'll save money by preparing your own food and eating at home.

8. Don't fill up on chips!

   a. You've probably tried just about every food available in America by now.

   b. At a meal, choose the foods you really want to eat; don't mindlessly eat the chips and bread set before you.

   c. Choose high-quality, tasty foods that you really want to eat. You don't have to eat everything available to you at one meal.

9. Eat three meals a day.

   a. Don't try to starve yourself or skip meals. You'll end up stuffing yourself with unhealthy snack foods.

10. Snacks are OK.

    a. Snack on unlimited amounts of fresh fruits and veggies.

    b. A few nuts are also OK for a snack.

    c. Keep plenty of peeled fresh fruits sitting on the countertop for snacks. Most people will go for the fruit if it's sitting right in front of them, ready to be eaten.

Epilogue

To err is human, to forgive [thyself] is divine.

In the last few weeks of writing *The Farmhouse Diet*, I am facing the reality that I have grown lazy and complacent. I have regained weight that I fought so hard to lose, slacked off on exercise, and backslid into old habits. But rereading and studying *The Farmhouse Diet* reminds me of what I need to do, what I can do. Rather than feeling depressed about my weight and lack of discipline, I am now encouraged that I can make those changes again to regain health and fitness.

So I have started over again by first reclaiming my goal weight and fitness as outlined in chapter 10. My ultimate goal is to lose twenty pounds, to go for a run of four to six miles at least four times per week, to drink less craft beer, to substitute additional vegetables for simple carbs at mealtimes, and to have dessert only once per week. Second, I have worked through Phase 1 including "Shake That Boost" and am working on Phase 2 of the Farmhouse Diet. Third, I'm really looking forward to Phase 3.

To optimize my chances for success, careful planning has been key. I weigh myself three times per week, exercise three to four times per week, and constantly remind myself of the weight-loss techniques I've learned in *The Farmhouse Diet*. I hold myself accountable by writing down my goals and keeping track of what I eat using the food diary from chapter 4. But even in this effort to rectify my past failings, I still sometimes fail. For example, I ate dessert twice this week, drank a craft beer instead of light beer last night, and missed several days of exercise last month due to an ice storm.

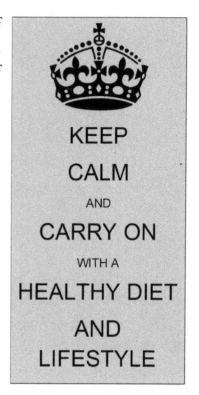

KEEP CALM AND CARRY ON WITH A HEALTHY DIET AND LIFESTYLE

So far, I have lost ten pounds since getting back on track and am back to a vigorous exercise routine. But should I feel guilty for failing to live up to the advice that I give to patients and am promoting in *The Farmhouse Diet*? After reflecting on this question, I have concluded that the answer is no. Why? Because I am just like you. I fail at times and am victorious at times. I often struggle to maintain good habits and beneficial lifestyle changes. That is, I'm human. I know that I will fail again, but I take comfort in knowing that I can make my way back.

My hope for you, the reader, is that you will be able to replicate the long-term success that I have had despite periodic setbacks and failures. If *The Farmhouse Diet* proves useful to you, and especially if it transforms your lifestyle, please pass it on to other fellow humans.

Weight-Loss Surgery and Nonsurgical Weight-Loss Devices

For many of us, dieting and exercise with concomitant lifestyle changes are not enough to produce the level of weight loss necessary to achieve good health. Whereas highly successful diets may result in a sustained 10 percent of total body weight lost (so if you weigh two hundred pounds, you can expect to lose and keep off twenty pounds), weight-loss surgery results in weight loss of 50 to 70 percent of excess weight (so if you are one hundred pounds overweight, expect to lose and keep off seventy pounds). This chapter describes in detail the different types of weight-loss, or bariatric, surgery, as well as nonsurgical devices and advanced technology. Also important to cover is the criteria for bariatric surgery so that you can make an informed decision regarding whether bariatric surgery is right for you. One important principle of bariatric surgery and nonsurgical weight-loss devices is that there is an inversely proportional continuum of how much weight one loses versus risk. In other words, the greater the weight loss, the higher the risk. The lesser the risk, the lesser the weight loss.

Bariatric surgery is not a crutch. Bariatric surgery is not radical. People are not "dying" to be thin. Bariatric surgery is not for the weak. Bariatric surgery is not an easy way out. Bariatric surgery is for those who want to take control of their lives and health. It's a means of achieving your goal of health. If excess weight were not a problem per se—that is, if it did not cause health problems such as diabetes, high blood pressure, sleep apnea, and crippling arthritis—then there would be no need for weight loss. Bariatric surgery requires hard work, perseverance, and commitment.

The definition of morbid obesity and the criteria for bariatric surgery and other nonsurgical weight-loss devices are based on body mass index (BMI), not actual weight. A better tool may be based on body-fat composition and distribution, but the technology to calculate those values is not widely available. Thus, the generally accepted method across the globe remains BMI.

BMI is calculated by dividing one's weight in kilograms by one's height in meters squared ($kg/[m]^2$). Making the calculation using pounds and inches simply requires a conversion factor, but in the age of smartphones and apps, I recommend plugging your weight and height into a BMI calculator. An app or website, such as the National Institutes of Health (http://www.nhlbi.nih.gov), is very helpful. Newer digital scales can also calculate your BMI.

Comorbidities of morbid obesity include sleep apnea, diabetes, high blood pressure, heart disease, fatty liver, lymphedema, severe acid reflux refractory to medications, pseudotumor cerebri, and polycystic ovary syndrome. You don't necessarily need medical comorbidities to have bariatric surgery, except when on the lower end of BMI.

There are no absolute upper or lower cutoffs for age, but certainly, advanced age puts one at higher risk. Few centers will accept septuagenarians, and accepting octogenarians is exceedingly rare. Patients under the age of eighteen years old would be treated as pediatric patients. Most pediatric patients are older, well-developed teens. Performing bariatric surgery in patients under the age of fourteen years is almost unheard of. Certainly, the child must have undergone adolescence. Expect special pediatric and psychological evaluations.

Other requirements include smoking cessation, previous diligent attempts to lose weight, no untreated or out-of-control medical problems, evaluation and counseling by a dietitian, and often evaluation by a psychologist.

When measuring the results of bariatric surgery, bariatric surgeons discuss them in terms of "excess weight loss": that is, how much weight above your ideal weight you would lose. So, if one is one hundred pounds overweight, and the surgery results in 70 percent excess weight lost, then one would lose seventy pounds; if one is one hundred forty pounds overweight, then if one lost 70 percent of excess weight, that would be about one hundred pounds.

CRITERIA FOR BARIATRIC SURGERY

BMI of 35+ (BMI of 30 to 35 requires obesity-related comorbidities.)

Age eighteen to seventies (Children under eighteen years should be treated through an adolescent program.)

Failed previous attempts at dieting

Nonsmoker

Ability to understand the dramatic diet and lifestyle changes that will occur

Note that these criteria are guidelines and will vary from program to program, among different insurance carriers, and even between different nationally recognized health organizations and advocacy groups.

Insurance

Specific criteria will vary based on the program you select. Also note that medical criteria are not the same as insurance criteria. In general, the insurance criteria are much more restrictive and onerous than the medical criteria. However, just because your insurance will not cover it does not mean that bariatric surgery is not important for your health. Many insurance carriers require patients to undergo three, six, or even twelve months of physician-supervised dieting. Some may require one to lose 10 percent of one's body weight prior to approval. Many insurance carriers require a three- to five-year history of morbid obesity, with documentation of yearly weights by a physician (some will accept dated photographs in lieu of weight documentation by a physician). If these insurance criteria seem burdensome, unfair, and perhaps even capricious, that's because they are. These criteria are not designed to make the results of bariatric surgery better but are put up as a barrier to prevent patients from getting surgery.

If insurance puts up roadblocks that would prevent you from getting surgery, remember that it is not because they know what's best for you. It is because they are trying to reduce the amount of money they spend on you. Even though the cost curves for bariatric surgery versus continued expenditures on health conditions that would be cured or ameliorated by bariatric surgery converge between two and three years, the insurance companies do not have the foresight that patients and physicians have. Because patients in this country tend to change employers and insurance carriers every few years, insurance carriers do not want to spend money so that the next company can then save money. This lack of rational, evidence-based health care only serves to drive costs up and increase the disease burdens secondary to obesity in the United States.

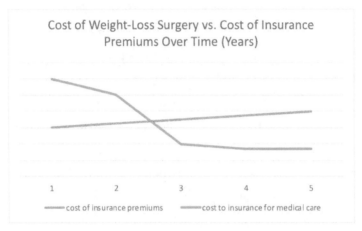

Figure A1-1. *Converging cost curves surgery vs. insurance*

In general, health insurance does not cover medical dieting or even dietary and nutritional counseling. There may be exceptions for weight-loss drug clinics run by obesity medicine specialists. However, many, if not most, will cover dietary counseling in patients with diabetes if it is provided by a special diabetes nutritionist. (It's very difficult for a dietitian to get this certification, so most patients with diabetes do not actually have access to this valuable service.) Remember that even though your health insurance may not cover bariatric surgery, it may still be important for your health.

Laparoscopic Surgery

Close to 99 percent of all bariatric surgery is performed laparoscopically. This means that the operation is performed using tiny incisions through which "trocars" or "ports" are placed. Thin instruments, such as needle holders, graspers, scissors, and staplers, are introduced through these ports. Visualization is via a long, thin camera that projects the image of the operation on a screen. It's easy to record these operations, so many of them have been posted on the internet. Because an old-fashioned big incision is avoided, pain is significantly less and recovery time is dramatically shorter with laparoscopic surgery.

Another mode of performing laparoscopic surgery is via a robot. Robotic arms are controlled by the surgeon at a console away from the operative field. The surgery is not performed by a robot, nor is there currently any artificial intelligence at work. That is still the stuff of science fiction. The surgeon actively controls the robot in real time while assistants are at the operating table. The instruments used in robotic surgery are basically the same as those in conventional laparoscopic surgery, just controlled differently. For the patient, there is no real advantage of robotic bariatric surgery over conventional laparoscopic bariatric surgery.

Laparoscopic Sleeve Gastrectomy

I describe this operation, also known as "the sleeve," first because it is currently the number-one bariatric surgery in America—indeed, the whole world—by numbers performed. The sleeve, also called the vertical sleeve gastrectomy, is generally a quick surgery performed laparoscopically. Expect a speedy recovery. Most patients are discharged from the hospital in a day or two, some in less that a day.

The sleeve surgery involves removing 85 to 90 percent of the volume of the stomach, including the floppy portion, or fundus, which holds most of the food. The part that pumps food out of the stomach, the antrum, is left mostly intact. Food still passes from the esophagus to the new thin stomach, then to the intestine, including the first part, called the duodenum. The sleeve is crafted with permanent, inert titanium staples. If one were to fill up the stomach with food, it would hold about three ounces. However, the sleeve functions mostly as a thin conduit for sending food down to the intestine. This slows down the transit time of food and thicker liquids, resulting in restriction of how much one can eat. You could think of it as a thin pipe about the diameter of your index finger. In addition to slowing down your eating and limiting the total amount of food you can eat, the sleeve also has metabolic effects that induce weight loss. Levels of ghrelin, the hunger hormone, decrease dramatically in patients with a sleeve. Patients lose about 60 to 70 percent of their excess weight over a year or less.

Laparoscopic Gastric Bypass

The gastric bypass, or "Roux-en-Y," has been performed for decades. Initially, the number of patients worldwide having a gastric bypass was low, but that all changed with the advent of the laparoscopic approach in 1994 by Dr. Alan Wittgrove in California. Since that time, almost all bariatric procedures are performed using this minimally invasive approach.

With the gastric bypass, your stomach is not removed as with the sleeve. It's bypassed. A small pouch is created out of the top of the stomach, and a limb of intestine called the roux limb is created. This limb of intestine is sewn or stapled to the pouch. Food then flows through the pouch into this limb of intestine. Although food does not go into the bypassed stomach, the stomach still secretes acid and mucous. Pancreatic digestive juices, as well as bile from the liver, flow down to join the roux limb. The mixing of food and digestive juices results in the absorption of nutrients. Because the first portion of the intestine, the duodenum, is also bypassed, there is an increase in the risk of vitamin and mineral deficiencies. The duodenum is very important for nutrient absorption, especially iron and calcium. When it is bypassed, other parts of the intestine take over most of this function.

In addition to slowing down eating and limiting the total amount of food you can eat, the gastric bypass also has metabolic effects that induce weight loss. Levels of ghrelin, the hunger hormone, decrease dramatically in patients who've had a gastric bypass. Patients lose about 70 percent of their excess weight over a year or less.

The mini-gastric bypass, loop gastric bypass, and single-anastomosis gastric bypass are significant variations of the standard laparoscopic gastric bypass but are not necessarily approved procedures and therefore cannot be recommended at this time. The Fobi pouch is just a technical variation of the standard laparoscopic gastric bypass, with no substantial differences.

Laparoscopic Adjustable Gastric Banding

Currently, the Lap-Band is the only adjustable gastric band available in the United States, where it has been available since 2001. Millions have been placed worldwide, but this surgery has become less popular since the advent of the laparoscopic sleeve gastrectomy. It is performed as a quick outpatient surgery. The adjustable gastric band works by restricting how much one can eat and controlling hunger. There is no malabsorption component. The band consists of a ring with an inner balloon that squeezes the upper stomach, just below the esophagus, tighter when fluid is added. Fluid is injected into the titanium and plastic port deep underneath the skin, then travels through the tubing to the band itself. Unlike the gastric bypass and the gastric sleeve, ghrelin increases after the band, much like what happens when one goes on a diet or is starving.

Frequent adjustments are critical for successful weight loss. Adjustments are not another operation but are similar to getting a shot. Generally, the first adjustment is done under x-ray guidance to maximize that fill. Subsequent adjustments, which are done about every month for the first year, are done either under x-ray or in the office.

The laparoscopic adjustable gastric band results in the loss of about 50 percent of excess weight over two to three years. The fastest weight loss is in the first year. One may lose weight quickly in the weeks immediately after band placement but then plateau until the optimal adjustment can be achieved. After that, adjustments are performed when gradual weight loss ceases or one becomes hungry. The goal is one to two pounds lost every week. One will never get to the perfect adjustment; ongoing adjustment will be necessary. To maintain weight loss, one needs to have the band adjusted every one to two years at a minimum. Also, proactive follow-up with the surgeon and having annual checks of the position and tightness of the band under x-ray will help prevent or delay problems with the band, such as slipping out of position or eroding into the stomach, and dilation of the esophagus. One of the band components, such as the inner balloon, tubing, or port, may eventually break, meaning it will not stay adjusted properly. If it is not properly adjusted, the patient will regain weight. Like any implantable device, it will eventually need replacing.

Currently, about 1 percent of bariatric operations nationwide use the laparoscopic adjustable gastric band, but it definitely still has its place in our armamentarium for treating morbid obesity.

Duodenal Switch

One way to think of this surgery is that it's like a gastric bypass and gastric sleeve combined. Most of the stomach is removed, as with the sleeve operation, and the duodenum is bypassed. The sleeve is attached to a limb of intestine, but most of the intestine is also bypassed. It works mainly by malabsorption, but it also restricts how much one can eat. This operation has powerful metabolic effects.

So, if one bariatric operation is good, then why not have two combined? The reason is that although the switch has the greatest percentage of excess weight lost, it is also the riskiest of the options. Most patients lose 85 percent or more of their excess weight, and it has the highest rate of cure of diabetes and other metabolic diseases. The surgery is routinely performed laparoscopically. Surgeons and their patients must remain more vigilant with medical compliance and follow-up than with other bariatric operations. Vitamin deficiencies and malnutrition, which can be devastating, are a much higher risk for patients who've had the duodenal switch than for other bariatric patients. The risks persist for a lifetime. Although some bariatric surgeons are rabid fans of the switch, I don't recommend it for first-time bariatric patients because, in my opinion, the risks are not worth the potential benefits.

Vagal Blocking

Vagal blocking is a fascinating new technology that took many years to develop. Currently, vBloc is the only vagal-blocking device approved by the US Food and Drug Administration (FDA) for weight loss. It works by blocking signals from the vagus nerve, thereby making one less hungry. In this laparoscopic surgery, tiny electronic leads are placed around the vagus nerves, which are dissected out by the surgeon where the esophagus meets the stomach. These leads trail through the abdominal wall to a generator implanted in one's abdominal wall or flank. The generator is about the size of a smartphone and wirelessly recharges nightly, the way an Apple Watch recharges.

Unfortunately, the results of the vBloc are disappointing compared to the hype surrounding it. Patients only lose about 20 percent of their excess weight. And the vBloc is subject to the same limitations as any implantable device, in that it will not last a lifetime. If the vBloc surgery entails the same level of surgical detail, risk, and maintenance as a laparoscopic adjustable gastric band, but the band results in significantly better weight loss, then perhaps it is better to get a band. Another consideration is the cost, which can be two to three times that of the laparoscopic adjustable gastric band or laparoscopic sleeve gastrectomy. Of course, what you pay is determined by insurance, so your out-of-pocket costs for any bariatric operation could be the same. Your insurance may cover the band, the sleeve, and the gastric bypass but not the vBloc.

Endo Sleeve

The endo sleeve is like a sleeve gastrectomy, but it is performed endo-scopically with a sophisticated suturing device. Unlike implantable devices such as intragastric balloons, this is real surgery. However, it's performed from the inside of the stomach, rather than using invasive ports through the abdominal wall under general anesthesia. Instead of removing the stomach, as in the laparoscopic sleeve gastrectomy, the stomach is rolled into itself to dramatically reduce the volume of food it can hold. There are no staples, and one's entire stomach is still present. The endo sleeve procedure is not risk-free, but it *may* carry a lower risk than the laparoscopic sleeve gastrectomy. Certainly, it carries a higher risk than an intragastric balloon. The weight loss is less than with the sleeve, perhaps less than with a laparoscopic adjustable gastric band, and usually more than with intragastric balloons. The very limited one-year data are promising, but the odds are that the sutures will break down and the stomach will unfold and go back to its original size. Currently, this may be a procedure for which the risks and monetary costs are not worth the relatively disappointing long-term weight loss compared with a sleeve or even a band.

Nonsurgical Weight-Loss Devices

Nonsurgical weight-loss devices are generally placed via an endoscope and/or removed under sedation. Although they do not involve surgery, they have potential risks. In general, they are safer than surgery and result in less weight loss. All but one are temporary. Most of these procedures are not covered by insurance, but there is considerable variation in coverage around the country. Some insurance carriers consider these procedures investigational. Another major consideration is that some of these devices are very new and have not been in existence long enough to measure long-term results.

Aspire Assist

This is a device inserted endoscopically through the mouth. This is more like surgery than intragastric balloons. A tube comes out of one's stomach to the skin, although the only thing you will see is a "button" that is well hidden by clothing. After eating a meal, which is to be eaten slowly, with lots of chewing, a tube is inserted into the button. A pump, which is small enough to fit inside a purse, is hooked up to the tube and sucks out semiliquid food, which is then emptied into a toilet. About one-third of the meal is aspirated out of your stomach. Could this be considered a socially acceptable form of bulimia? Maybe, but obese patients are more interested in healthy solutions than old taboos. I was highly skeptical of this device at first, but the results are fairly good. Unlike other nonsurgical weight-loss devices, it should be regarded as permanent.

Intragastric Balloons

Currently, there are two FDA-approved intragastric balloons on the market, but more are in the developmental pipeline. They differ in how they are placed and the contents within the balloon. All are placed nonsurgically (no scars), and all are temporary. Although the excess weight loss with intragastric balloons is significantly less than with bariatric surgery, the risks are also greatly reduced. The FDA indications for intragastric balloons are patients with a BMI between 30 and 40 and no prior gastric surgery.

Orbera is a spherical saline-filled balloon about the size of a large grapefruit; it weighs over two pounds when filled with saline. It is placed endoscopically under sedation or general anesthesia and removed in a similar manner six months after implantation. Saline-filled balloons work by occupying space, delaying emptying of food out of the stomach so that you feel fuller longer, and stretching the baroreceptors of the stomach. Nausea and acid reflux are common symptoms, which are mitigated with medications. These balloons result in weight loss of approximately 25 percent of excess weight at the time of removal. Weight regain is common.

The Obalon intragastric balloon system consists of three oblong, air-filled balloons about the size of an orange. Each balloon is placed by swallowing a large capsule under imaging guidance; then, each is inflated with air via a thin catheter that trails out of the mouth. The catheter is immediately and easily removed from the mouth. This is repeated twice a few weeks after the initial balloon placement for all three balloons. When examined under x-ray, the stomach looks like it is filled with balloons. All three balloons are removed at six months endoscopically under sedation. Obalon works by occupying space in the stomach and reducing hunger. It results in less weight loss than the saline-filled balloons, about ten pounds less, but has virtually no symptoms of nausea or acid reflux.

I think of intragastric balloons as a boost to a sensible diet. They are tools that increase weight loss. For maximum weight loss with an intragastric balloon, it's critical that one follows a healthy diet, such as the Farmhouse Diet, for the duration of balloon placement as well as after the balloons are removed. Lifestyle changes are critical. Otherwise, one would certainly regain the lost weight.

Intestinal Liners

Currently, these are investigational and not yet ready for prime time. They are temporary and work by blocking the absorption of nutrients. The risk profile, such as causing bowel obstruction or nutritional deficiencies, may end up limiting the applicability of this technology.

Is Bariatric Surgery the Right Answer for Me?

Bariatric surgery and nonsurgical weight-loss devices are not magic, although it may seem like it. The magic may start to fade after a few years. It's hard work, not only to get the surgery but also to adapt to and maintain a healthy lifestyle in the years that follow. Taking multivitamins and calcium, seeing your bariatric surgeon and dietitian, and getting lab work annually are keys to long-term success. Some patients need additional vitamins, such as B12 and D, or other nutritional supplements.

Attending a bariatric support group has been shown to help patients keep weight off. Exercise and sticking to the bariatric diet are essential, just as with all diets and any healthy lifestyle change. Although losing weight and sustaining weight loss are most ideally achieved through diet, bariatric surgery could be just what the doctor ordered.

If you believe that bariatric surgery or a nonsurgical weight-loss device is right for you, hopefully this chapter has armed you with the information that you need to make a wise choice. There is not a one-size-fits-all approach to bariatric surgery. Fortunately, there are lots of tools to aid you in the battle against obesity.

RISKS OF BARIATRIC SURGERY

The short-term risks of bariatric surgery are less than 1 percent for serious complications at most accredited programs across the world. There are also long-term risks to consider, such as vitamin deficiencies and malnutrition. Dying from bariatric surgery is exceedingly rare compared with other major operations, and the risk of death should certainly be much less than 1 percent. Risks vary by procedure. I like to think of procedures on a continuum of risk as well as weight loss (and improvement of health). For example, the bypass is riskier than the sleeve, which is riskier than the band. But the bypass leads to greater weight loss and improvement in health than the band. The duodenal switch is the bariatric operation with the highest risk. The different intragastric balloons are generally regarded as the lowest-risk procedures. The risks of other nonsurgical devices and procedures are harder to pin down and highly dependent on the level of experience of the program where they are performed. You will want to choose an accredited program to minimize your risks of surgery, as well as ask your surgeon what her or his individual complication rates are.

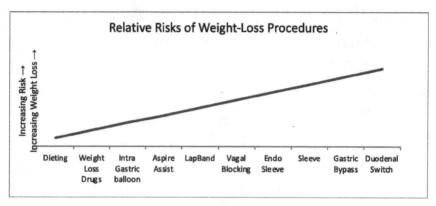

Figure A1-2. *Risks of weight-loss procedures*

APPENDIX 2

The Seven Habits of Highly Effective Dieting

1. Fresh fruits and veggies.
   a. Avoid processed or canned vegetables and casseroles.
   b. You can have unlimited quantities—don't worry about calories.
   c. Nuts and seeds are not considered fresh fruits or veggies.
2. No fried, greasy, or oily foods.
   a. Chips, fries, fried chicken and fish, fried burgers, doughnuts, and so forth are off-limits.
   b. Watch oily and high-fat salad dressings.
3. No processed foods.
   a. No snack foods.
   b. No TV dinners, microwave meals, and so forth.
4. Whole grains and complex carbs are good.
   a. Avoid simple sugars and simple carbs, such as anything with potatoes, cornmeal or corn sugar, or added sugar. That includes sweets and desserts.
   b. Choose whole-grain pasta.
   c. Carefully select stone-ground whole-wheat breads.
   d. Choose grains such as buckwheat, barley, quinoa, and so forth.

5. Dairy, cheese, and eggs are good for you.
    a. Yes, you can eat an egg.
    b. Watch the fat content in cheese and milk.
    c. Full-fat yogurt is good for you.
    d. There's no such thing as diet ice cream.
6. Fats are OK.
    a. Make sure, however, that fat is not the foundation of your diet.
    b. Lean meats are generally better, but you can have beef, pork, chicken, and fish.
    c. Certain oils, such as extra-virgin olive oil, are healthier than others.
7. Occasional "naughty" treats are OK.
    a. Avoid sugary beverages because they can contribute quite a few empty calories to your diet.
    b. Occasional desserts are OK, but they should be a treat, not a part of every meal.
    c. Alcohol, including beer and wine, is OK . . . again, in moderation.
    d. You can have bread with a meal. Just don't make it the whole meal.

Strategies for Dieting Success

1. Eat and cook at home.
   a. Avoid eating out. Most restaurants have very limited healthy eating options.
   b. Foods at restaurants almost always have much higher fat, carb, sugar, salt, and calorie counts than the equivalent food that you would cook at home.
   c. Don't know how to cook? Give it a try—it's actually fun!
2. Don't keep the "bad stuff" in the house.
   a. Even though it may be there for the kids, I guarantee that eventually you'll get into it.
   b. Keep fresh fruit sitting out on the counter to snack on instead of the bad stuff.
3. Keep engaged, active, and busy.
   a. Boredom leads to mindless snacking.
4. Read nutritional labels.
   a. The packaging and ads can be deceptive.
5. Artificial sweeteners are OK if they aid in compliance and reduce cheating.
   a. There are often gastrointestinal side effects of artificial sweeteners.
   b. The use of artificial sweeteners may prevent you from kicking your sugar addiction.

6. Stop eating when you start to feel full.
   a. Many people have the habit of stuffing themselves, especially during holidays.
7. You don't have to buy more expensive "organic" or gluten-free foods.
   a. Eating healthier can be more expensive, but you don't have to shop at an expensive specialty store to get healthy food.
   b. You'll save money by preparing your own food and eating at home.
8. Don't fill up on chips!
   a. You've probably tried just about every food available in America by now.
   b. At a meal, choose the foods you really want to eat; don't mindlessly eat the chips and bread set before you.
   c. Choose high-quality, tasty foods that you really want to eat. You don't have to eat everything available to you at one meal.
9. Eat three meals a day.
   a. Don't try to starve yourself or skip meals. You'll end up stuffing yourself with unhealthy snack foods.
10. Snacks are OK.
    a. Snack on unlimited amounts of fresh fruits and veggies.
    b. A few nuts are also OK for a snack.
    c. Keep plenty of peeled fresh fruits sitting on the countertop for snacks. Most people will go for the fruit if it's sitting right in front of them, ready to be eaten.

Endnotes

Chapter 1
Figure 1-1: The author's great-great-grandparents, Dr. Henry F. and Mrs. Arbana Gilliland. Circa 1900.

Figure 1-2: Craig M. Hales, Margaret D. Carroll, Cheryl D. Fryar, and Cynthia L. Ogden, "Prevalence of Obesity and Severe Obesity among Adults: United States, 2017–2018," *NCHS Data Brief*, no. 360 (Hyattsville, MD: National Center for Health Statistics, 2020).

Figure 1-4: Karen R. Flórez, Tamara Dubowitz, Naomi Saito, Guilherme Borges, and Joshua Breslau, "Mexico-United States Migration and the Prevalence of Obesity: A Transnational Perspective," *Archives of Internal Medicine* 172, no. 22 (2012): 1760–62.

Figure 1-6: Parvez Hossain, Bisher Kawar, and Meguid El Nahas, "Obesity and Diabetes in the Developing World—A Growing Challenge," *New England Journal of Medicine*, 356 (2007): 213–15.

Figure 1-7: Berkeley Food Pyramid, BFP Creation and Design, Co-Creators Michael Corbett, Mary Hardy, Scott McCreary, and Renee Robin. Graphic Design by Noreen Rei Fukumori.

Chapter 3
Photos and art in chapter 3 licensed from Adobe Stock.

Chapter 6
Figure 6-1: Source US Food and Drug Administration.

Special Note: Unless otherwise cited, all other photographs, figures, and graphs in *The Farmhouse Diet* are produced by the author or used by permission of the patient.

About the Author

A native of Alabama, Wm. Jay Suggs, MD, FACS, FASMBS, FFSMB, returned home after his general surgery training at the Mayo Clinic and bariatric surgery fellowship in Princeton, New Jersey, to start his first bariatric surgery Center of Excellence. Dr. Suggs is a board-certified surgeon and is also a fellow of the American College of Surgeons and a fellow 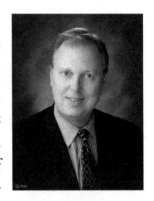 of the American Society for Metabolic and Bariatric Surgery. He has degrees in biology and chemistry from Emory University and earned his medical degree from the University of Alabama at Birmingham. Dr. Suggs and his wife and three daughters live in Decatur, Alabama, where they are an active part of their community.

Writing, lecturing, and teaching have always been passions of Dr. Suggs. He is an associate professor of surgery and director of medical education at his regional medical center. He has been involved in the leadership of multiple professional organizations and hospitals, including serving on his state's medical board and the state board of health.

Dr. Suggs is the president of Alabama Bariatrics and has performed more than three thousand bariatric operations, including the laparoscopic sleeve gastrectomy, the laparoscopic gastric bypass, the laparoscopic adjustable gastric band, intragastric balloons, and bariatric revision/redo surgery.